T0229875

Contemporary Psychodrama

Contemporary Psychodrama weaves together psychodrama and psycho-analysis with illustrative clinical examples, whilst preserving the essence of psychodramatic philosophy and methodology. Previously unavailable in the English language, this book presents José Fonseca's diverse new approaches to psychodrama together with a blending of theories.

The book is divided into clear sections, covering:

- New approaches to psychodrama theory
- New approaches to psychodrama technique
- Psychodrama and sexuality
- The past and future of psychodrama

Fonseca's innovative ideas include the adaptation of techniques originally intended for groups to individual psychodramatic psychotherapy. He distinguishes between not only the normal and the mentally ill but the normal and the optimal, and presents a detailed developmental psychology, inspired by Moreno and Buber, but clearly influenced by object relations theory.

Contemporary Psychodrama presents the original concepts of a leading light of the Brazilian psychodrama movement that will be of great benefit to all professionals working with psychodrama.

José Fonseca, M.D., Ph.D., was one of the pioneers of the psychodramatic movement in Brazil and a founder of the Brazilian Federation of Psychodrama.

Contemporary Psychodrama

New approaches to theory and technique

José Fonseca

Translations by Julia Carleton Pinelo and Elizabeth Walden Tambor

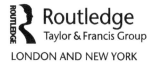

Routledge
Taylor & Francis Group

LONDON AND NEW YORK

Published 2004 by Routledge
27 Church Road, Hove, East Sussex BN3 2FA

Simultaneously published in the USA and Canada
by Routledge
711 Third Avenue, New York, NY 10017

Routledge is an imprint of the Taylor & Francis Group, an informa business

Copyright © 2004 José Fonseca

Typeset in Times by Mayhew Typesetting, Rhayader, Powys

British Library Cataloguing in Publication Data
A catalogue record for this book is available from the British Library

Library of Congress Cataloging-in-Publication Data
Fonseca Jose, 1965–
    Contemporary psychodrama : new approaches to theory and
technique / Jose Fonseca. – 1st ed.
        p. cm.
Includes bibliographical references and index.
    ISBN 1-58391-988-0 (hardback)
    1. Psychodrama. I. Title.

    RC489.P7F657 2004
    616.89'1523–dc21

                                                    2003015998

ISBN 978-1-58391-988-0 (hbk)

To Maria, of course

Contents

Foreword

José Fonseca has managed to accomplish many things with the publication of this series of papers in English. He helps overcome the inordinate discontinuity between psychodynamic and psychodramatic theory. The total separation of these two psychological systems has had the result of marginalizing the profession of psychodrama from the rest of psychotherapy, resulting in insufficient training of psychodramatists in psychodynamics and leaving no point of access for most therapists to reconcile the natural appeal of psychodrama with their scientific orientation.

Classical psychoanalytic theory, based on libido theory, was an attempt to account for the whole richness of mental life as copious branching out of sexual energy. More recent analysts have reformulated these views, substituting the idea of human relationships themselves as the central feature of mental life. The relational schools such as those of the ego psychologists, the interpersonalists and others have arisen and influenced psychoanalysis from within. On the other side, psychodrama was founded on the base of Moreno's sociometry. This latter has suffered from the criticism that it diminished the role of the individual human psyche to a simple this or that role of preference for one person over another. Sociometry was about group patterns rather than about the structure of the human mind. Fonseca shows that just as a computer can generate very complex patterns on the basis of zero vs. one choices, so can the human mind. The results of our many and internalized sociometric interpersonal choices is what makes us who we are. Thus Moreno's sociometry can blend naturally with the relational schools of psychoanalysis and psychodrama, even more so.

Fonseca presents a detailed developmental psychology, explicitly based on Moreno and Buber but clearly influenced by object relations theory. Fonseca is crystal clear here, as he breaks the developmental phases down into detailed sub-phases – all of great importance. The reader will be grateful for his simple, clarifying diagrams. He then carries these ideas in a rather unexpected direction. The medical model distinguishes between the sick and the well; a person either has tuberculosis or does not. If one does not, there is nothing better. But this way of understanding of physical health is not applicable to mental life. Fonseca distinguishes not only between the normal and the subnormal (mentally ill) but between the normal and the optimal. For example, the capacity for Moreno's role reversal is seen as a *sine qua non* of mental health. Therefore, he speculates that there must be a maximum degree to which this capacity extends. This maximum, which he equates with Buber's I–Thou relation and Moreno's encounter, is invested with an almost mystical intensity. Similarly, Fonseca focuses on the tele–transference relationship rather than on the transference alone as is usual. He understands transference to refer to those aspects of the patient's perception of the therapist which are distorted by internal untransformed past relations in contrast to the actual features of the therapist. Moreno's "tele" is the undistorted part. In considering the patient's perception of the therapist, the conventional psychodynamic therapist confines their patient's attention to the transference. But Fonseca does not consign the tele simply to the rest of the patient's experience of the therapist that is left over (i.e. not transferential). He sees the accurate perception of the other as a complex and subtle process which can be raised to a high art, the ability to read minute non-verbal cues, etc. It is also the function of therapy to maximize this capacity for the patient.

Fonseca includes a vivid review of the history of the Morenos's twenty-year struggle to found the International Group Psychotherapy Association, not simply as their personal triumph but of the coming to be of group psychotherapy as a permanent and vital entity in the world.

James M. Sacks

Acknowledgements

I would like to thank Anne Ancelin Schützenberger, who encouraged me to publish this text and recommended the Brunner-Routledge editor Joanne Forshaw, and her reviewers, who offered many wise suggestions on both the composition and the content of the chapters; James M. Sacks who, besides writing a most worthy foreword, demonstrated his kindness once again; Sandra Rocha da Cruz and Mariana Kawazoe who provided the essential work on the structure of the book (typing, researching original citations, etc.); and Liz Walden Tambor and Julia Carleton Pinelo, especially the latter who translated the majority of the book, for their competence and friendship.

José Fonseca

Introduction
Trying to cross the language barrier

In 1961, J. L. Moreno, in the preface to the Spanish language edition of his book *Psychodrama – First Volume*, commented that Latin culture was fertile ground for the development of psychodrama. Indeed, the psychodramatic movement has spread considerably in Argentina and Brazil over the past forty years. In Brazil, where Portuguese is spoken, there are approximately 4,000 people working with psychodrama. But it is important to remember that Brazil is a continental country with more than 8 million square kilometers and 175 million inhabitants. There are also more than a hundred books on psychodrama written by Brazilian authors. Despite this strong representation, Brazilian psychodrama is almost unknown to the rest of the world for a simple reason: we do not speak or write in English, the "Esperanto" of our time. So, the only way of crossing this language barrier is to translate our texts into English. For this reason, I have put together some articles, translated at different times and circumstances, in the hope of being heard by my colleagues on the other side of the ocean.

The following texts have been organized with a didactic objective, but it is also perfectly possible to read them in whatever order the reader should choose.

In Part 1, I have put together some texts that I hope will contribute to the study of psychodrama theory. Just as in order to understand the socio-economic and political culture of one country it is necessary to study those of other countries, in order to really understand a psychological theory it is important to know others. Dialogue with other references broadens one's consciousness of the limits of any given theory. In assimilating ideas from other schools of thought I have attempted not to lose the main line of psychodrama theory (that is, socionomics), which is fundamentally relational, in the hopes of preserving its essence.

The first two chapters of Part 2 represent an attempt to make psychodramatic techniques more flexible, so that they can be utilized in individual psychotherapy. Despite the fact that classical psychodrama is eminently focused on group work, Moreno is open (though, in truth, timidly) to its utilization in an individual context (monodrama). The proposal behind both *relationship psychotherapy* and *internal psychodrama* is to bring psychodramatic technique to the foreground in individual procedures. Also within this section of the book the reader will find *theater-psychodrama*, a way of utilizing the theater as a warm-up to later psychodramatic action, and a report on the Open Sessions that have been held weekly in São Paulo for some twenty years.

The challenge of addressing how psychodrama approaches sexuality, along with some Morenian reflections on my clinical practice, led me to write the four texts that comprise Part 3. They clearly do not represent, however, any official psychodramatic view on sexuality, but merely the view of one psychodramatist on the theme.

Lastly, in Part 4 the reader will find a text that relates Moreno's – or better, the Morenos's (as his wife Zerka contributed extensively to the project) – struggle to found an international organization for group psychotherapy. It was his wish that all group therapists be united in one place to exchange experiences. In the next chapter there is an analysis of the scientific paradigms that have guided medicine, psychology, psychoanalysis and psychodrama in the past century. I try to show that J. L. Moreno was a visionary, in the sense of one who has a vision – a pre-vision – of the future.

Obviously, I am not the only representative of the Brazilian psychodramatic movement, but this will give you at least some idea of our way of thinking and working with psychodrama.

José Fonseca

Part 1

New approaches to psychodrama theory

Chapter 1

Scheme of human development (inspired by Moreno and Buber)

An approach to sanity and insanity*

This text combines the theories of Moreno and Buber with my experiences from clinical practice, which includes experiments carried out in a psychodramatic psychotherapy group, composed mostly of psychotics.

Bowlby's (1958) studies on "attachment" corroborate many of the affirmations made here. He offers a firm basis for the interpersonal theories I describe and for the foundation of "a relationship psychotherapy" – by which I mean psychotherapy which takes into account, as a technical procedure, the two-way (as opposed to unilateral) interaction established between patient and therapist.

Role reversal as a "measure"

From a practical perspective, a correlation between Buber and Moreno would have to begin with *the encounter*, the *I–Thou* (from hereon referred to as the *I–you*), their greatest point of convergence. Buber refers to role reversal (the psychodrama theory and technique) as "experiencing the other side", an essential condition for the *I–you* encounter. Moreno's concept of role reversal represents the culmination of a development process (of the matrix of identity) in the human being. Hence, by means of the psychodramatic technique of role reversal ("experiencing the other side") we would have the necessary tool for a practical study of Buber and Moreno. In other words, with the capacity "to reverse roles/experience the other", we have the possibility for the encounter. Either allows us to see that a

---

* This is the first part of Chapter V, Psychodramatic Study of Madness, from the book *Psychodrama of Madness: Correlations Between Moreno and Buber* (São Paulo, Ágora, 1980 [5th edition, 1999]). The book is divided into five chapters: I: J. L. Moreno and the Psychodramatic Theory; II: M. Buber and Dialogic Philosophy; III: The Encounter – Buber and Moreno; IV: The Genesis of the Encounter: Hasidism; and V: Psychodramatic Study of Madness. Although this is only a fragment of the whole, I believe that the reader will not have any difficulties in understanding it if already familiar with Moreno or Buber.

healthy person has the potential and capacity for the encounter since they would be capable of "reversing" or "experiencing the other".

Through psychodrama and the technique of role reversal, the capacity to "reverse with or experience the other" can be measured. As such, one would be measuring the degree of health or sickness afflicting a person. Laing (1973) suggests that sanity or psychosis may be tested by the unity or disunity between two people. Role reversal proposes the same or goes even further. For Moreno (1977), personality begins to form with the development of roles. So, to study the personality formation, given the strict relationship between the "role process" and its formation, he presents "the role test" (1977, p. 161).

Acting out a role always suggests the presence of "another". For each role there is a complementary role or counter-role. The relationship (mother–son, doctor–patient, etc.) emerges from the meeting of the two. Role and counter-role are "co-existent", "co-acting", "co-dependent" (Moreno, 1977). The presence of a great number of psychotic elements (during an outbreak or severe regression) in a personality would correspond to a total inability to play and reverse roles. Likewise, the total absence of psychotic elements (the ideal model) would result in a perfect role-reversal performance. Between these extremes lie the myriad variations. The "sign of not reversing roles", means some healthy process has been altered. This is in agreement with Moreno's theory of the development of the matrix of identity (see diagram on p. 22), where, in regressive order, we would first have the "loss of role reversal". Alteration of the intermediate phases would then take place, followed by the inability to perform one's own role (recognition of I) leading to "indifferentiation". An alteration in the ability to reverse roles would be the first indication of "sickness".

It is important to note that a patient's capacity to reverse roles is not established in a single psychodramatic scene but throughout numerous scenes. First of all, the protagonist must be appropriately warmed up for the scene. Then, only by observing a series of psychodramatic sessions can one conclude to what point the patient is unable to reverse particular roles, a specific role, several roles, or all roles. Such observation permits one to confirm whether blocks in an emotional sector pertain only to a particular relationship, or if the block is more extensive or even global.

Neurotics[1] are frequently incapable of performing in the role of the other. Roles, which contain strong emotional stress, lead to restricted spontaneity and performance. For example, in presenting a great inner conflict with a particular person in the psychodramatic scene, the person is unable to perform the role. The psychotic's block, especially during an

---

1 The nosography utilized is anterior to the DSM.

outbreak or with "defects of personality", is much more profound and intense, making role reversal a threatening experience.

Patients with processual evolution and consequent "defects" in chronicity are also unable to role reverse. However, when the personality is "conserved", outside the psychotic episodes, it may be possible. I have observed that in the remission phases of cyclical psychosis patients manage reversal. Yet, in remission from schizophrenic outbreaks role reversal may be more difficult, depending on the intensity of the "defects". With psychogenetic and/or reactive psychosis, the ability to reverse roles returns with the disappearance of the psychotic symptoms. Neurotics, or non-psychotics, including character neurosis or psychopathies, manage a considerably better performance of roles and role reversals, despite blocks sometimes existing for particular roles and for reversals. In short, the more sickness afflicting the personality, the greater the difficulty in playing and reversing roles – both in psychodrama and in life.

J. L. Moreno mentions (1975) that role reversal should be used carefully when a poorly structured individual is involved, especially when the other participant is a well-structured individual. For example, "double technique is the most important therapy for lonely people . . . A lonely child, like a schizophrenic patient, may never be able to do a role reversal but he will accept a double" (J. L. Moreno, 1975, p. 157). Precisely as one would expect, since the double stage corresponds to stages before the development of role reversal.

Referring to the Rojas-Bermudez (1975) role diagram, in neurotics the "self" would expand, hindering performance of the complementary role. In his own role, the individual would act according to stereotypes of all the neurotic conflicts accumulated during his life. The thought that this neurotically crystallized role or type of linkage could be transformed would generate panic. Thus, a block would exist for certain roles. In the psychotic, once something has set off this "alarm", a highly expanded "self" would emerge as a supposed defense. In more severe cases expansion would disguise all vital roles, making connection with complementary roles difficult, if not impossible. Attempts to make contact are inhibited by this "self" barrier, perceived as threats of invasion and loss of boundaries (in patients in psychotic outbreaks and/or with "handicapped" personalities).

Mazieres (1970) states that in the psychotic patient the sequence would be: (a) alarm signal; (b) threat of being invaded and destroyed; (c) expansion of "self" as defense (covering up the roles) and; (d) difficulty or impossibility in performing roles (with role-to-role relationships there are no linkages). I add that, without linkages, the psychotic would find him/herself deprived of the *you* – alone in psychotic solitude.

J. L. Moreno (1975) states that human beings suffer fundamentally from the incapacity to realize all the roles that are part of them. They are always greater than their undertakings show, and this greatness is also the reason for their misery. Anguish arises from the pressure exerted by all these inadequately performed roles, roles that are repressed and demanding realization. In the psychotic, it is as if pressure and anguish are at a maximum. Under such pressure, the psychotic frequently explodes, performing megalomaniac and grandiose roles, as if to compensate for a long period of restriction. The resulting delirious roles are a rebellion against personality repressing procedures that hinder the free flow of forbidden roles.

Paths between reality and fantasy

The psychotic, unable to distinguish fantasy from reality, regresses. According to Moreno (1977, p. 114) in "The Breach Between Fantasy and Reality Experience", a child's development is accomplished through two preparatory processes – one related to real acts, the other to fantasy acts. The problem is not one of leaving the world of fantasy in favor of the world of reality, which is practically impossible. Rather, it lies in creating the means to enable the individual to master both situations, able to shift from one to the other. Nobody can live forever in a totally real world, nor in a totally imaginary one. The psychotic is blocked on the pathways that allow free transit between the two worlds and thus confuses them. He/she, therefore, has difficulty in getting out of him/herself – of being *the other* – of performing at the level of the "as if", of the "make believe", of fantasy. It might seem strange that, being in the realm of (pathological) fantasy, the psychotic is unable to interpret a scene's (psychodramatic) fantasy, dominated instead by a "fantastic rigidity". The psychotic cannot reach the free path, the healthy exchange between the two worlds (as occurs to a greater or lesser degree in all psychotic patients).

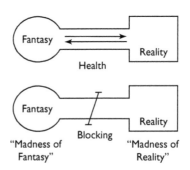

Likewise, remaining exclusively in the realm of reality would be a "realistic rigidity", a madness, "the madness of reality". Henry Miller, in his magnificent essay on Rimbaud, says that the last desperate attempt to flee from madness is to become so completely wholesome that one does not realize one is mad: "Rimbaud never lost touch with reality, conversely, he held on to it like a maniac; what he did was abandon the true reality of his being" (1968, p. 112).

In these cases, the "tele" (Moreno) is altered. Psychotics are unable to grasp the surrounding world. Psychotics are unable to act, to get out of themselves and seek the other (Buber and Moreno). They submerge themselves in their transferential world.

A case study from group psychotherapy may illustrate the point: Joana, 28 years old, looked bored and annoyedly aloof. She was ostensibly indifferent to the environment, distrustful, introverted, inhibited, with schizoid retraction and a reduction of her "vital contact with reality" (Minkowsky, 1961). Her thought sequences seemed poor, clouded by continued fantasy. Some ideas were overvalued, compromising experiences. In the group, she would not state her opinion about the others when asked to, making personal complaints instead. She was unable to perform complementary roles during dramatizations, and found it extremely difficult to transfer herself to fantasy. Yet, whenever she did manage to, she had difficulty coming back to reality. On one occasion, during a group scene of a shipwreck, she removed the watch of one of the shipwrecked persons (played by an auxiliary ego). After the scene was over, and even after the end of the session, she refused to return the watch, arguing with elements from her "as if" role played in the dramatized scene. During another session, she performed with an auxiliary ego who played the role of a homosexual. Since then, she has always considered him to be homosexual.

Her inability to be the "other" during fantasy play and its mixture with reality, together with her inadequate emotional level, gives us an idea of the existential weakness and self-loss of existence.

The impossibility of being the other, the *you*, of performing and reversing roles according to Moreno, corresponds to the incapacity to experience or include the other side according to Buber. Under such conditions there is no capacity for mutuality and reciprocity. These patients find themselves mute to spell out the "basic words". According to Moreno and Buber, this would be the failure of the *encounter*. Both conceive of man as the bearer of cosmic linkages and the cosmos as the great cradle of human beings. Since, for Moreno, man develops from the cosmos (through the matrix of identity) and, for Buber, man starts his evolution through the "basic words", then Moreno's "indifferentiation" phases correspond to Buber's innate *I–Thou*. Through Moreno's "role reversal" and Buber's "experiencing the other", man becomes fit for *encounter*, for a full "dialogical" relationship.

A scheme of human development

Performing the "role of the other" is not something that comes about suddenly and fully fashioned. It requires a whole sequence of developmental stages that overlap and frequently operate jointly. For Moreno, the matrix of identity – comprised of five stages – is a child's first emotional learning process. The first stage is characterized by the child's inability to distinguish himself from his/her environment – he/she feels him/herself as one with the rest of the world ("oneness"). The second stage is characterized by the infant centering attention upon *the other* and his/her bewilderment, discomfort and curiosity in discovering he/she is not, in fact, one with the world. In the third stage, the child separates *the other* more completely from him/herself. In the fourth, the child is able to perform the role of *the other*. During the fifth stage, identity reversal is complete; the child is able to play the role of a third person who, in turn, performs the child's role. Obviously, the last two stages do not occur in the early months. These stages of infantile development are the psychological basis for all role-performing processes. Starting at the extreme of indifferentiation, gradually the child will begin to concentrate on the opposite extreme and reverse roles with the other.

These three stages could be simplified to: (1) the total identification of the *I* with the *you*, of the individual with everything that surrounds him/her ("oneness"); (2) the recognition of the *I* with his/her peculiarities as a person; and, finally, (3) the recognition of *you*, the acknowledgement of others and of the world.

The scheme, which follows, though based on Moreno and Buber, has also been influenced by other authors. It has been modified to include several additional stages not included in the outline described above. The conclusions are based primarily on clinical reflection, not on the direct study of children.

Indifferentiation

It is important to state that, for both authors, the human being is considered a cosmic being, coming from and returning to the cosmos. The cosmos is a human cradle in birth and death.

Pregnancy, gestation and birth is a grandiose process for three beings – father, mother and child. But, due to biological factors, the child is in closest communication with the mother. When a newborn baby nurses, the baby and the mother (the first auxiliary ego) are both intensely engaged in the same act.

During the nursing period, the mother is relatively independent from the child. She leaves, then returns when further nurturing is required. From this point of view, the *I-mother* is somewhat disconnected from the *you-child* (not withstanding the strong affective union). This is not the case with the child. The *I-child* confuses itself with the *you-mother* as the distinction between the two has not yet emerged. The child mixes its things with those of the surrounding world. The child's and mother's elements are one. The child experiences all objects and people coexistentially ("complete spon-taneous all-identity"). According to Spitz (1966), this is the indifferentiation stage, the pre-object state. This "co-existence, co-action and co-experience" illustrates the relationship between the child and the world in the primary stage of Moreno's (1977) "matrix of identity".

During this stage, the child is governed by internal mechanisms. When the child is cold, hungry or in pain, he cries, and "the world" takes care of him. The child is mixed with the world, resting in his cosmic cradle. The child does not distinguish between the *I* and *you* (you-person, or you-object). Schematically, the *I* is represented in this stage by an oval con-figuration where the *I* and *you* are mingled, confused.

$$\boxed{\begin{array}{c} \text{You} \mid \text{You} \mid \\ \text{I} \quad \mid \quad \text{I} \; \text{You} \mid \text{You} \end{array}}$$

In this stage, a child cannot survive alone, as do animals of some other species. The child requires someone to take care of him, an auxiliary ego (mother, nurse) – somebody who will do what the child is unable to do, somebody who understands what he desires. It is quite common for the mother's sixth sense (tele) to detect certain conditions in the child that others fail to perceive. Of course, this does not mean the overprotection of certain mothers who act out their own anxieties (transference) in their children. The mother, severed from the baby by childbirth, continues in close communication as the child's auxiliary-ego or double.

It is exactly this stage of cosmic identity that is applied as a theoretical basis for the psychodramatic *double technique*, where the function of the auxiliary ego is to express the thoughts and feelings that the protagonist does not perceive or is unable to express, providing conscious and/or unconscious support. In a broader sense, the *double principle* governs all psychodramatic work, insofar as the psychodramatist (director or support-ego) always functions as an auxiliary ego. The protagonist is the "child" in need, looking for something he/she cannot find alone. This "child" desires the aid of somebody who understands him/her (tele), and provides the means to find what he/she seeks. However, psychodramatists should not merely give what they think the protagonist requires (counter-transfer), but should, through sensitivity and appropriate techniques, facilitate the protagonist's self-exploration.

As an example, during a psychodramatic session, a delirious young man accepts a double performed by an auxiliary ego to whom he has become highly attuned. When the auxiliary ego is no longer the double (leaving the patient's side and sitting elsewhere in the room) the patient cries out, "so now it's two against one again!" The close harmony he felt with the double fostered a sense of unity with the self.

Symbiosis

As the child develops, this experiencing of cosmic identity attenuates itself. The child is striving to acquire an identity as an individual person, to discriminate the *other*, the *you* and the world. But he does not yet fully manage to do so. Thus, we find the child still united with the mother by a strong link.

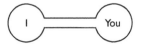

The persistence of this union–link, or its non-definitive disconnection, might generate distinctive traits in both the child's future adult personality and behavior toward the world. This stage is also governed by the *double principle*. If there is any link remaining, if the psychological "umbilical cord" has not been cut, a full personal identity cannot be found. At this stage, a communication deficiency, a pathology in the *inter* between the *I* and the *you*, could be disastrous. Alternation in the communication, the *inter*, exists because both elements are directly involved in the union. Just as the child depends on his/her mother, she depends – psychologically – on the child. The "atmosphere", the "flow" between the *I* (child) and the *you* (mother), will have major significance in structuring the *I* and will establish the shapes and patterns of future relationships.

Recognition of the I

The child now enters the period of recognizing him/herself, of discovering his/her own identity. The child is polarized by him/herself. At the somatic level, this is the period when the child starts to become aware of his/her own body in the world. The child realizes that his/her body (him/herself) is separate from the mother (*you*), from people and from objects. He/she begins to distinguish and identify bodily sensations, such as hunger and pain, and slowly becomes aware of his/her physiology – ingesting, defecating, breathing, sleeping, being awake and urinating (psychosomatic roles).

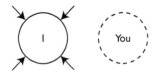

Slowly this process of self-recognition becomes more sensitive, preparing the child to differentiate proximity/distance, gentle/aggressive touching, relationship/solitude, etc.

At an earlier stage, a child in front of a mirror does not recognize him/herself: he/she is the baby, indefinite. Later on, the child becomes aware that the image is him/herself. He/she recognizes him/herself. The child begins to perform his/her own role; he/she exists as an individual, as if he/she were the center of the world. A child, still unaware of him/herself as a person, uses the third person (he/she) to refer to him/herself. This stage corresponds to the *recognition of I* or *mirror stage*, which, in reality, is always present in a person's life. This first stage (or peak) – early childhood – is both fundamental and the most important. The second peak is adolescence, and the third is the passage to senility. Man is forever involved in this unending, unfailing, process of self-learning for which psychotherapy can serve as a useful aid.

This stage is the theoretical foundation for the psychodramatic *mirror technique* which Lacan (1971) describes as greatly significant to the formation of the personality. The psychodramatic *mirror* is a procedure aimed at enabling the protagonist to see him/herself through the performance of his/her role by the auxiliary ego. It is my opinion that the *mirror stage* is also the theoretical foundation for the *soliloquy technique*, which is nothing more than a conversation with oneself, the possibility of seeing oneself in a relationship. In any given relationship, there is a moment in which the individual can become "remote" and reflect upon his/her way of relating, both upon the other and upon the relationship itself.

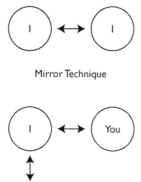

Mirror Technique

Soliloquy Technique

Recognition of the you

A distinction between the *recognition of the I* and the *recognition of the you* is made for purely didactic reasons. They are really part of the same process. At the same time that one is becoming aware of oneself as a person, one is also engaged in perceiving the other, entering in contact with the world, identifying the *you*. The child is "polarized" by the *you*, magnetically drawn – as if in centrifugal movement – to the world outside him/her.

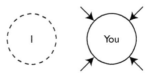

It is common to find a child "pondering" an object – examining it, discovering it. This same behavior is frequently seen when the child discovers another's body, comparing his/her own anatomy with that of another, reflecting upon and asking about the differences. It is during this stage of discovery that the *other* feels and reacts to the child's initiative. For instance, if the child hits a friend, the friend may cry or react aggressively. This process of learning about the *other* is extremely important for the establishment of satisfactory relationships in the future.

"Corridor" relationships

In this stage, the I and the *you* are recognized. Here, says Moreno, the "breach between fantasy and reality" is established. The child acquires the capacity to distinguish between fantasy and reality, between what *I* am and what "the rest of the world" is.

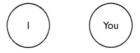

The first rehearsals of role reversal that will formally substantiate themselves later on are played out here.

Emotional and cognitive capacities are perfected. The child gets acquainted with the other *you(s)* in his life. *You*, therefore, does not mean only the mother. There is a *you* at every step forward. The child forms "corridor relationships" – exclusive and possessive relationships. The child is identified as an individual. He/she differentiates him/herself from the other, but feels that the *you* exists only for him/her, a natural reflection of his/her recent past, when the child felt as one with the *you*. He/she denies the possibility of his/her *you* relating to others.

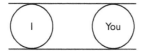

Corridor relationships

The child has not yet grasped the world and the relationships of the people around him/her as a whole. He/she has not internalized the family's sociometry – in gestalt terms. He/she feels unique, central.

Pre-reversal

At a certain stage, the child initiates the role reversal process. This process takes shape from the time he/she initially performs his/her role (role of the *I*) in the world, and then plays the role of the other (the *you*) – playing other people, animals and objects. Sometimes the child pretends to be a puppy, a thief, a doctor, etc. He/she plays the *you* role but without reversal, without reciprocity. However, we soon observe that in the child's playful environment of discovery, he/she starts to rehearse role reversal when, for example, the girl's doll is she herself and the girl is the doll's mother, or she is her baby brother's mother, and so on.

This is not yet an egalitarian way of reversing roles, but rather a protected training toward this end. Directly after this stage, the child will accomplish full role reversal, but without the reciprocity and mutuality that comes with full maturity.

Parents usually know that children perform this role reversal with pleasure, spontaneously. Quite often, these reversals become enjoyable games between parent and child. Both J. L. Moreno (1975) and Z. T. Moreno (1975) took advantage of their son Jonathan's natural role-reversal period to study development at this stage.

However, I think that this process attains its full development only in adult life. For a fully accomplished role reversal, the child has to go through other phases. Therefore, I call the initiation of this stage the "pre-reversal period", to distinguish it from its complete development. The completion of this stage would also signify the apex of the person's *telic* development, which a child has not yet reached.

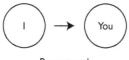

Pre-reversal

I utilize this diagram to show that the process is not finished, or synchronized, as it will be later in life.

Triangulation

"The triangulation crisis" corresponds to Freud's Oedipal stage (1968). I use the term "triangulation crisis"[2] to enhance the communicative aspect of a previously bipersonal relationship that has now become triadic, playing down, but not denying, the sexual aspect that varies with culture and time.

Imagine the child forming his "corridor" relationships (with the mother, the father, etc.), vacillating in reversals (pre-reversal) and at a given moment realizing that he/she is not unique to his *you*: there is a *she/he* also present.

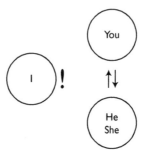

There is a *he/she* related to its *you*. It is as if the child has lost his/her *you*, as if he/she has been deprived. The child may respond to this critical, destitute situation with a good or bad resolution of the triangular complex, depending on the intercommunication between the three. We cannot comment on the child's health or sickness, but on the sanity or pathology of this triadic, sociometric communication. All the relationships in question are of major significance.

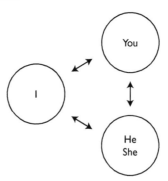

The relationship *I–you* is directly dependent on the *you–he/she, I–he/she*, and so forth relationships. To understand these dynamics, one could

2 The expression "triangulation" is also used by Rojas-Bermudez (1978): "The triangular type of relationship is the base of socialization."

imagine three people holding hands and moving freely. Each individual is related to the other two. The three are bound by the same commitment.

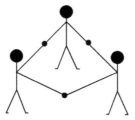

The ideal solution to this "triangulation crisis" would be the child's acceptance that the *others* have relationships that do not depend on him/her and that this does not necessarily imply a threat of affective loss (the child is not wounded). The child might substantiate linkages with the *you* (*I–you*); he/she might relate with the *he/she*, which at this moment is a *you* (*I–he/she*); or the child can accept the *you–he/she* as an independent relationship. A "gestalt-like" relationship with the *you–he/she* couple is possible.

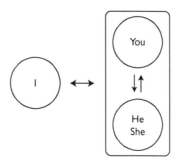

Circularization

Once the child has gone through the triangular stage of development, he/she is ready to relate to more people (more than two or three) simultaneously. The "circularization stage" occurs when the child begins to have contact with groups, friends, school, etc. This corresponds to the child's "socialization".

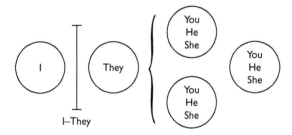

Using again the image of people holding hands, we now have four people:

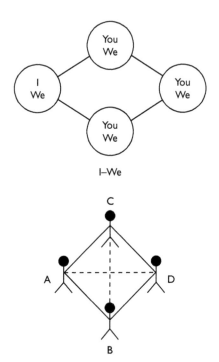

Unlike the triangular situation, where three elements communicate on equal terms in three direct relationships, in this quadrangular situation there is a significant change insofar as there are four direct relationships and two indirect ones (A–D and B–C). That is, the quadrangle contains four people yet has six relationships. If the set were composed of five people, there would be nine relationships. Considering that the relationships between each element could contain attraction, refusal, or indifference (as Moreno proposes), these sets would become increasingly complex.

Thus, the circularization stage represents the initiation of the human being to the sociometric experience of groups.

In going through the stages of bipersonal and triangular relationships, the individual acquires the capacity to relate to the *they* and, later, to also feel as part of a group or community, which allows him/her to penetrate the world of the *we*. The possibility for group "inclusion" – to feel the warm involvement of the *I–we* instead of the coldness of the *I–they* – is an important step toward the individual's satisfactory future group and social relationships.

Role reversal

Following all this role-play "training" (the child plays the *I*, the *you*, the *he/she*, the *they* and the *we*), the individual will attain the full capacity for human relationships of reciprocity and mutuality. The "role reversal" stage, the theoretical foundation for the psychodramatic technique bearing its name, then occurs.

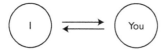

Role reversal signifies "including" oneself on the other side and vice-versa, as Buber states. It means that A and B – *I* and *you* – are both present and able to captivate each other with corresponding exchanges of positions. There is the possibility for real and profound communication between the two people. As the individual acquires the capacity to place him/herself in the other's position and permits the other in his/her position, he/she acquires a better knowledge of the reality of other personal worlds and, as a result, of his/her own as well.

The role-reversal stage is the concrete manifestation of the *tele*. This is the apex of the *tele*'s development. One could correctly say that reaching the role-reversal stage is a sign of maturity and psychological health. One might further argue that, very often, it is by means of the psychodramatic technique of role reversal that one can detect the total transferential burden that the *I* loads on the *you*: the *I* relates to itself, to its own internalized images, not with a real *you*.

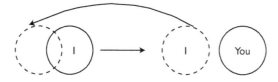

Transference

A transferential relationship is a relationship between the *I* and its own inner ghosts. A transferential relationship is not a *telic* one; it is a diseased linkage, not a healthy one. I believe that the role-reversal stage begins very early, around the second or third year of life, and reaches its peak in adult life.

This process is developed (or practiced) precisely through the reversal of real roles that the individual experiences during his/her life. Psychodrama presents an adequate setting for protected training. The inability to reverse roles in adult life signifies severed communication with the *you* in the current scene. The psychotherapist must certify if this incapacity concerns a particular *you*, or several *yous*, or if this incapacity is broader, as with psychotics.

Encounter

In the ideal situation – total capacity to reverse roles – both Moreno and Buber suggest that there is a special moment known as the *encounter*. The encounter happens so abruptly and so intensely that *spontaneity/creativity* is released through an act of mutual surrender (the surrender principle). This is an "insane" moment, yet represents the moment of "health" in a relationship. It implies a vital orgasm, expressed by the explosion of "divine sparks" in the fraction of time in which this loss of personal, temporal, and spatial identity occurs.

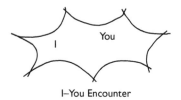

I–You Encounter

The people involved fuse in a cosmic reunion. The *encounter* is a reconnection with the cosmos through the (latent) cosmic elements that all human beings carry within them. It is a return to one's origins.

People encompassed in this cosmic encounter short-circuit later recover their own identities, strengthened and revived. The *I* will be more *I* and the *you* more *you*.

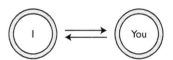

One might say that cosmic revival is similar to an individual's first experiences in the maternal womb and in the first months of life as previously described. But there is a qualitative and quantitative difference. One is the shelter, peace, and rest within one's origins; the other is a fleeting, but unforgettable, moment of a greater communicational ecstasy with oneself, the other and the universe. However, the essence of both experiences is the same, the cosmic element being the common denominator. The climax of development is similar to one's beginning. End and beginning unite. Extremes meet. One enters the realm of the dialectic of opposites.

One might ask if these moments of *encounter* occur frequently. I recall Herman Hesse's "Magical Theatre. Entrance only for the odd . . . only for the mad" (1969, p. 28). If the capacity to fully reverse roles implies the individual's (ideal) psychological maturity, the total and unrestricted possibility for such an encounter would be the privilege of a God: a man-God.

A continuation of the moment of *encounter*, a journey without return, represents the entrance into the realm of madness. Just as a health climax would be a moment of insanity, persistence of health would be madness. This is one aspect of cosmic balance and harmony.

I believe that these aspects of "unity and duality" – via Buber and Moreno – stem directly from Hasidism and the cabala. These concepts are also related to oriental philosophies such as Taoism. Weil (1973) explains that the circle represents an absolute where the Yin and the Yang are not separated by hermetic divisions. There is a constant transfer from one state to the other. There is always positive in the negative and negative in the positive, holiness in the sinner, sin in the saint, etc. This system of unity/duality, madness/sanity applies to the scheme where sanity and madness are adjacent and similar, yet distinct.

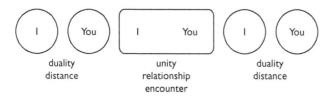

The distinction between "health" and "sickness" is a question of path, orientation and direction. Some seek "health", through "reversal/experiencing the other", and through the *encounter* reach cosmic revival. Others seek it regressively. People also look for the cosmos, but in the opposite direction. This would correspond to my image of "health/mental disease", through Buber and Moreno.

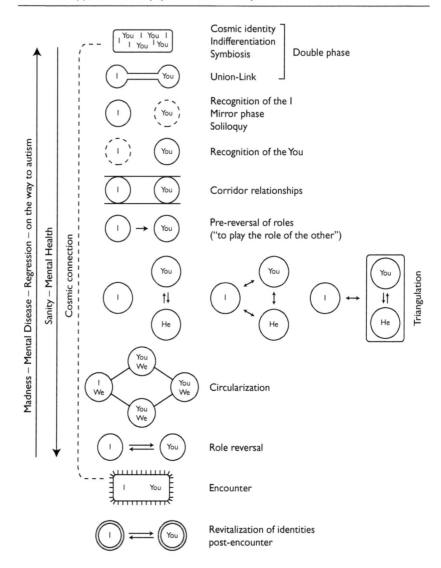

Development of the human being – Health–Disease

"Role reversal/experiencing the other" can serve as a method for evaluating the personality. The full capacity for "reversal/experiencing the other" (*telic* capacity) represents ideal health, while the incapacity to do so would be the opposite: disease. Transference is a failed *encounter*. Thus, the technique of role reversal could be used to "measure" a person's degree of "sickness-disease".

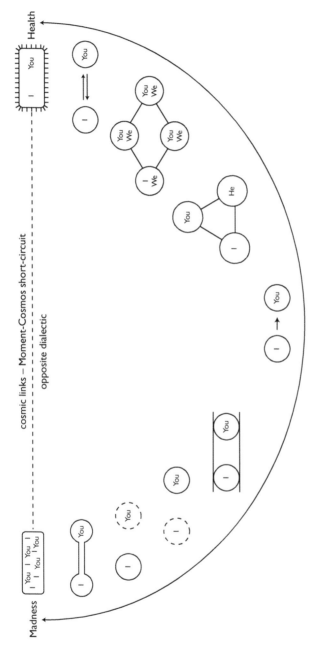

The circular setting of the diagram gives clear evidence of the proximity between sanity and madness and their dialectic liaison (opposite)

The circular setting of the diagram is similar to a diagram by Cooper (1971) also dealing with "normality". Normality is equidistant from "madness" and "health".

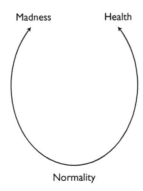

Psychotics, largely impotent for the *I–you*, are isolated in previous stages (see diagrams). In the despair of their "*I-istic*" solitude, they create a delirious-hallucinatory *you* to accompany them. People in an outbreak, in psychotic phases, or affected by psychotic conditions for a long time have regressed and/or fixated at earlier stages of development. Although unable to attain reversal, they still remain "individualized" or "personalized". The greatest regression (disaggregation, autism) corresponds to the first stage – experiencing the sensation of total unity with the mother and the world. Here, the loss of individualization or depersonalization occurs.

Neurotics already exhibit blocks, difficulties or conflicts in relating to specific *yous*; consequently, they have difficulties in realistically, *telically* "reversing/experiencing the other", without transference or projection. Certain peculiar ways of linking, added to specific characteristics of the search for the *I–you* shaped during the development process, form different personality types. As previously discussed, pathologic anxiety is a distortion of the ontological desire for the *encounter*. This anguish could hasten an artificial and uncontrolled quest for the *encounter*. "Anxiety is cosmic; fear is situational. Anxiety is provoked by a cosmic hunger to maintain identity with the entire universe" (J. L. Moreno, 1975, p. 154). In this way, a drug addict tries to enhance the brilliancy of the anticipated moment with drugs. Hysterical manifestations are pseudo-relationships intended to fill the void of a true relationship. Phobic expressions signify imprisonment in the desire/fear encounter circle. Obsessive aspects represent a shield of systematic control over the environment, trying to reach the *I–you* through rationalization and intellectualization. Psychopathic traits correspond to the individual's action against a world that frustrates him/her "dialogically", in an attempt to make it responsible for his/her failure.

Mental disease could also be seen as an *encounter* pathology of the *I–you*. It is a sickness located in the *I–you*, or, better, "between" the *I* and the *you*, a distortion of the *inter*, a pathology of human communication. In fact, an *I* alone is an abstraction since the *I* only exists insofar as it encounters the *you*. The *I* only acknowledges and lives in its world when it manages to interact with a real *you*. The *I* hungers for the *you*. The supreme goal is "reversal" and the *encounter*. Buber, in his preface to the psychiatrist Hans Trub's book (preface transcribed in Friedman (1976, p. 191), states: "A soul is never sick alone, but always through a betweenness, a situation between it and another existing being." Laing (1973, p. 15) states that psychotics are unable to feel "together" with others or "at ease" in the world. On the contrary, they experience a desperate isolation. While studying "Peter's case" (pp. 132–148), he transcribes this patient's remark: "I was as if dead. I detached myself from the others and shut myself up within myself. And I perceive that when one acts like this, one dies up to a certain point. It is necessary to live in the world with the others. If this does not happen, something dies within yourself . . ."

In accordance with Martin Buber's "dialogic" philosophy, a psychiatrist might state that psychotics remain isolated in their disease because they are unable to find the *you* for their *I* or that they are unable to speak with a concrete *you*. The world becomes a projection of their *I*. They only manage "dialogue" with a fictitious *you*.

If Buber and Moreno were here, they might agree that humans, in their anguish for the *you*, for the *I–you*, for the *encounter*, for the "cosmos", for "God", sometimes sink into psychotic solitude. They desperately seek in delirium a substitute for their void.

References

Bowlby, J. (1958). The nature of the child's tie to his mother. *International Journal of Psychoanalysis*, 39: 350–373.

Buber, M. (1977). *Eu e tu*. São Paulo: Cortez e Moraes. (Original edition: *I and thou*. New York: Charles Scribner's Sons, 1970.)

Cooper, D. (1971). *Psiquiatria y antipsiquiatria*. Buenos Aires: Paidós. (Original edition: *Psychiatry and anti-psychiatry*. London: Tavistock Publications Ltd, 1967.)

Fonseca, J. (1972). *Correlações entre a teoria psicodramática de J. L. Moreno e a filosofia dialógica de M. Buber (Correlations between J. L. Moreno's psychodramatic theory and M. Buber's dialogical philosophy)*. São Paulo: Faculdade de Medicina, University of São Paulo, Doctoral Thesis.

Fonseca, J. (1977). El psicodrama y la psiquiatria – Moreno y la antipsiquiatria (Psychodrama and psychiatry – Moreno and anti-psychiatry). *Momento*, 3: 4–5.

Fonseca, J. (1980). *Psicodrama da loucura (Psychodrama of madness)*. São Paulo: Ágora (6th edition, 2003).

Freud, S. (1968). *Obras completas*. Madrid: Biblioteca Nueva. (English edition: *Complete works*).

Friedman, M. (1976). *Martin Buber: the life of dialogue*. Chicago: The University of Chicago Press.

Hesse, H. (1969). *O lobo da estepe*. Rio de Janeiro: Civilização Brasileira. (Original edition: *Der Steppenwolf*. Germany: Montagnola, 1951. English edition: *Steppenwolf*. Harmondsworth: Penguin Books, 1965.)

Lacan, J. (1971). Escritos. México: Siglo XXI. (Original edition: *Ecrits*. Paris: Seuil, 1966. English edition: *Ecrits. A selection*. Translated by Bruce Fink in collaboration with Héloise Fink and Russell Grigg. New York: W. W. Norton, 2002.)

Laing, R. D. (1973). *O eu dividido*. Petrópolis: Vozes. (Original edition: *The divided self*. London: Tavistock Publications, 1960.)

Mazieres, G. H. (1970). Incorporación del psicodrama como técnica en la psicoterapia grupal psicodramática con pacientes psicóticos cronicos (Incorporation of psychodrama as a psychodrama group therapy technique with chronic psychotic patients). *Cuadernos de Psicoterapia*, V, 2.

Miller, H. (1968). *O tempo dos assassinos*. Rio de Janeiro: Record. (Original edition: *The time of the assassins: a study of Rimbaud*. New York: New Directions, 1946, 1962.)

Minkowsky, B. (1961). *La esquizofrenia (Schizophrenia)*. Buenos Aires: Paidós.

Moreno, J. L. (1975). *Psychodrama: Foundations of Psychotherapy – Second Volume*. New York: Beacon House, Inc.

Moreno, J. L. (1977). *Psychodrama – First Volume* (5th edn). New York: Beacon House, Inc.

Moreno, Z. T. (1975). *Psicodrama de crianças*. Petrópolis: Vozes. (Original edition: *Psychodrama in the crib and psychodrama in a well baby clinic*. New York: Beacon House, Inc., 1958.)

Rojas-Bermudez, J. G. (1975). *Que es el psicodrama (What is psychodrama)*. Genitor: Buenos Aires.

Rojas-Bermudez, J. G. (1978). *Núcleo do eu (The nucleus of I)*. São Paulo: Natura.

Spitz, R. (1966). *El primer año de vida del niño*. Aguilar: Madrid. (Original edition: *The first year of life: a psycho analytic study of normal and deviant development of object relations*. New York: International Universities Press, Inc., 1965.)

Weil, P. (1973). *Esfinge. Estrutura e mistério do homem (Sphinx. The structure and mystery of man)*. Petrópolis: Vozes.

Chapter 2

Freud, Moreno and bossa nova

Elements of relationship psychology

Recently, after a conference at which I spoke, an attentive young participant approached me and asked what psychoanalytic theory I follow. I responded that I was a psychodramatist with psychodynamic orientation. I spent a few minutes more trying to explain that my method of psychotherapeutic work is the result of the combination of professional influences I have had. As I returned home I began considering this complex process of a psychotherapist's training, and what the main influences on me had been.

We are always under some influence or another. This may be a simple book, which we enjoyed, but afterwards forgot. Other influences, however, are profound and influence the course of our professional career. If we analyze the practical and theoretical influences of a professional we can better understand who he/she is and how he/she works. The greatest influence on a psychotherapist is his/her personality – the fruit of his/her genetic inheritance and environmental (family, education, culture) factors. However, this text is not meant to be a professional autobiography (and much less a personal one). It is restricted to an analysis of the primary theories which have influenced my career.

There are many authors that we read, but few who are *absorbed* into our professional universe. This *absorption* of influences is determined not only by intellectual conditions but also by affective aspects. There is conscious–unconscious identification with the author. When we like an author it is because he/she either exposes ideas that we have already had, or those that we have not yet had, or those that we begin to have upon reading his/her work. In this sense, the author functions as our alter ego, and when we like an author it is because we are "appreciating ourselves". In other words, the process of learning is directly connected to the narcissistic aspects of the personality, be they *telic* and/or *transferential*, where processes of sublimation, repression, projection, identification, etc., are included. All enthusiastic reading passes through the *telic–transferential* prism when we oscillate from passion to hatred for our authors. Commenting on one of Freud's works, Garcia-Roza (1993) notes that nobody reads what is written. He further states that Freud knew this, because he sought another text originating from the manifest text (using the reference to dreams) written by the unconscious. Or, more romantically, we could say that the authors we read are like the many people we know, few of whom ever truly enter our hearts.

Before I move on to discuss the principal points of this theme, I would like to consider a brief point about my professional roles – both roles that anchor and those that are anchored – which will help clarify my proposal. In chronological order, my professional roles have been that of doctor, psychiatrist, psychodynamic psychotherapist and psychodramatist. Medical texts are very objective in describing signs and symptoms, in diagnosing, and in therapeutic conduct. I believe that both the positive and negative influences of a medical background, allied with aspects of my personality, have made me opt toward direct and practical authors. I do not enjoy psychological ruminations, pompous interpretations, and sterile philosophies. This characteristic, perhaps, has influenced me in the search for objective, strategic, and action (not just verbal) methods. Psychotherapeutic processes that are exaggeratedly prolonged cause me to suspect that the main objective has been lost and that a reciprocal relationship neurosis has been established.

Here I will attempt to follow a spontaneous narrative, not necessarily following the chronological order of influences but rather organizing the text according to topics in order to facilitate the reader's comprehension.

Psychodrama and psychoanalysis

Psychoanalysis has been the primary influence in my role as psychotherapist. Let us distinguish Freud's psychoanalysis, because its ingenious creation became larger than Freud himself, from other "psychoanalyses". My psychoanalytic initiation occurred by way of Freudian dissidents. In my youth, while I was still studying medicine, I read two authors who were then in fashion: Karen Horney and Erich Fromm. Both of Germanic culture, they emigrated to the United States. They were a part of the so-called culturalist school. They valued social and cultural aspects of the human being, attenuating Freudian exaggerations (relative to child sexuality, penis envy, and the Oedipus complex, for example). When I began reading Freud directly I had already developed a certain critical base, even if I was naive at the time. Whether a result of this or not, the truth is that I always had more affinity for psychoanalytic authors, dissidents or otherwise, that emphasized the relational aspect of psychoanalysis: transference and counter-transference (*I–you*), Oedipal triangle (*I–he/she*) and narcissism (*I–I*). Among these authors I include Franz Alexander, Michael Balint, John Bowlby, Ralph Greenson, W. Ronald Fairbairn, Erik Erikson, Harry Stack Sullivan, Harry Guntrip, Heinz Kohut, Donald Winnicott and others.[1]

1 The majority of these authors were the object of study at the PSG (Psychodynamic Study Group) of the Daimon-CRS (Center for Relationship Studies), São Paulo.

Currently, accompanied by my worthy companions, I have taken on an inspired chronological reading and rereading of the Freudian, Kleinian and Bionian works at the PSG (Psychodynamic Study Group) of the Daimon-CRS (Center for Relationship Studies). As I read Freud, Klein and Bion, I transform them through the psychodramatic filter and express them through a relational psychology. You might say, in other words, that I do a psychodramatic reading of Freud's, Klein's and Bion's works.

Along these lines, I believe that it is useful to comment on some considerations in respect to psychodrama. What emerges as most important from Moreno, more than one specific concept, to me, is his relational philosophy. I read Moreno with enthusiasm because he was absolutely different from anything I had seen in psychiatry and traditional psychotherapy in the 1960s and 1970s, and he was sufficiently revolutionary to feed the soul, thirsting for freedom and transformation (in addition to everything else we lived through under a military dictatorship). One can be Morenian without ever pronouncing a single Morenian concept, as long as one's spirit remains alive. As I have indicated, I conceive of the Morenian concepts as unified. In this way, the *telic* phenomena are related to the *encounter* that occurs in a *moment*, with the liberation of *spontaneity*, which in turn leads to *creativity*. Tele–transference occurs in relationships established among roles (role and counter-role) that are connected through sociometric criteria. The roles and the tele–transference originate in the *matrix of identity*. This delineates Moreno's ideas about child development. The concept of the *matrix of identity* permits the contemporary psychodramatist, who also knows psychoanalysis, to fuse Morenian relational psychology with psychoanalytic psychodynamics. In this way, we have psychodynamic concepts which are delineated by a relational philosophy, within the spirit of Moreno's work, but which also bring contributions from psychoanalysis to the study of child development that Moreno's work does not include. Some Argentinian authors, such as Martinez Bouquet, Moccio and Pavlovsky (1971), and other French authors such as Lebovici, Diatkine and Kestemberg (1958) and Anzieu (1961) join psychodramatic and psychoanalytic concepts, whereas Schützenberger and Weil (1977) attempt a synthesis among Freud, Moreno, Kurt Lewin and others.

More recently, Paul Holmes (1996) has presented a correlation between psychodrama and the theory of object relations. I, too, attempt an integration of the theories. As I wrote in "Ainda sobre a matriz de identidade" ("More on the matrix of identity") (Fonseca, 1996a), I seek "fusion, just as musical fusions[2] exist, between the matrix of identity and relational psychoanalysis, attempting to preserve the psychodramatic language. Despite

---

2 I use the well-expressed term "fusion", employed by Lia Fukui, sociologist and psychodramatist, in the MSG (Moreno Study Group) – Daimon, to understand this fact.

the 'grandiloquence' (yet excusing myself for the pretension), bossa nova can be said to represent the influence of American music on samba, yet this does not mean that bossa nova is not Brazilian music." In this sense, this position cannot be understood as an eclecticism, which is a philosophic system *formed from elements collected from diverse sources without exclusively following one.* Here, one follows the psychodramatic system as a basis for incorporating psychodynamic–psychoanalytic concepts.

Relationship/separation

From these concepts, I began to develop the summarized perspective on human development that I present here. The fulcrum of this understanding is the relational psychosocio dynamic of the human being. Here, relationships from the *"matrix of identity"* are included, progressing from the primary intrafamilial relationships, where identity is formed, passing through the internalization of these relational models, and then coming to the exterior again, in the relationships of adult life.[3]

In discussing the relationship, the polar opposite, separation, is implicit. Between the two there is a gradation of experience that sets the tone for each relationship (or each relationship/separation). In child development, the relationship–separation dynamic is the basis of the personality formation. We shall see some elements of this process that were brilliantly studied by John Bowlby (1982). Despite, or perhaps due to, the fact that he was supervised by Melanie Klein, Bowlby is reserved toward her ideas, especially those which refer to the valuation of the internal world (internal conflicts between aggressive and libidinous impulses and the central value of envy in personality function) to the detriment of the importance of early-childhood internalization of relational models in forming the personality. Beginning in the 1960s Bowlby launched his trilogy, *Attachment, Separation and Loss*, in which, according to Montoro (1994), one of the Brazilian authorities on the subject,

> Classic psychoanalytic thought was turned upside down; he rejected the concepts of energy and impulse and the importance of orality and sexuality in child development; he attacked the concepts of fixation and regression; he adopted an evolutionary and ethological point of view to investigate human behavior; he proposed cybernetic models similar to those adopted in family therapy, he proposed an executive structure to substitute the Freudian concept of ego and created a new theory of defense mechanisms based on studies of information processing.
>
> (Montoro, 1994, p. 43)

---

3 The basic structure of these ideas can be found in Fonseca (1980, ch. 5).

I will try to show what Bowlby's literature inspired in me. I include some teachings within relational psychology, an approach that presents man as an eminently relational being. Direct observation demonstrates that a baby has a clear preference for proximity to people. The baby seeks not only nourishment but also, primarily, relationships. From the phase in which this search is indiscriminate and any relationship will do, the child begins to express preferences (primary sociometry), varying in intensity, in a demonstration of childlike "falling in love" with certain people in his/her world. Others, who are not included in this select group, are pushed away with crying and aggression. Gilda Montoro (1994, p. 45) emphasizes that what we can call "attachment behavior" is "all forms of behavior that have as an objective the obtaining or maintaining of proximity to another specific and preferred person, called the figure or object of attachment". While "learning" the relationship, the child is also "learning" separation. When a child is abandoned by one of these select people, a series of relationships are presented which we can divide, didactically, into four phases. In the first, when perceiving the initial signs of separation, the response is *anxiety/fear*. There is a manifestation of *anger* (aggression) due to the desire to stay in the relationship. What then follows is *sadness* from having experienced abandonment. The last phase, which we can call the *resolution phase*, or *defense formation*, corresponds to the return to the (at least, apparently) normal state, with the experience internalized. If, on the one hand, this cycle makes up the basic learning of relational life, on the other hand it opens up possibilities for the appearance of a varied range of defenses – *personality "techniques"*[4] (*hysteric, phobic, obsessive, schizoid, paranoid, etc.*) – against the pain of separation and loss. Bowlby calls these defenses "development paths". This group of psychological reactions indelibly influences the internal partial *I(s)* (as we shall see) that are forming during this period, giving origin to the primary and secondary personality traits. These steps in relationship–separation learning form the basic structure for all future affective relationships. The atmosphere of the relational field will be guided by feelings (love, hate, anxiety, guilt, sadness, happiness, jealousy, etc.) involved in the relationship–separation process. The result of these influences in the *matrix of identity* will mean, in the future, "relationally" secure or insecure adults (secure and anxious attachment, according to Bowlby).

We should consider, furthermore, that over this primary base of "learning" relationship–separation, the psychological development process continues. In "The Psychology of Becoming Ill" (Fonseca, 1989, chapter III), I discuss the superimposing of two periods of relationship/separation

---

4 Fairbairn (1975) employs the expression "technique" to describe the psychological resources that a child uses in the sense of structuring his/her personality.

"learning". One period deals with the incorporation of the self-value concept that governs self-esteem and the discriminative perception of the esteem that others dedicate to us. This phase corresponds to the narcissistic structuring of the personality. Based on the origin of the *ideal I*, the child oscillates between perceiving him/herself as the most beautiful, loved and powerful (relationship), and sensing him/herself as the ugliest, least loved and destitute of power (separation). The other period corresponds to triangulation, or the appearance of a third person in a formerly two-person relationship (e.g. mother/child relationship). The third person is the necessary facilitator in the learning of separation. In this way, the symbiotic egg is broken and the psychological birth of the baby (separation) takes place – the concretization of the identity. Triangulation, from this perspective, is a broad relational process that encompasses the Oedipus complex.

In Bowlby's observations about child development we find further important elements for comprehending the *telic* component in human relationships. Bowlby believes that children attach themselves more easily to adults who quickly respond to their stimuli (primarily crying), and who are evidently open to the relationship (playing, laughing, talking). In other words, a baby prefers sensitive people who show pleasure in the relationship. In psychodramatic words, we may say that the child "connects" to people who offer a more evident possibility of establishing a *telic* "click".

In the next section, I take a classic clinical case from psychoanalytic literature, "The Little Hans Case", from Freud (1976, pp. 15–154), to illustrate some of these ideas in a practical manner. We shall observe how the "relationship/separation" dynamic can be useful in the study of child development.

Relational focus of the little Hans case

First of all, it is worth noting an interesting historical-relational aspect among the participants of the case: Hans, his father, his mother, and Freud. The mother had been a patient of Freud's. Both she and her husband were admirers of Freud and decided to observe the psychological development of their son. The father began to take notes that he would then submit to "Herr Professor". These were received with pleasure, because Freud himself had not directly studied children, and his theoretical observations originated from adult treatment. The father was not interested in freely observing the psychological development of his son, but rather in proving psychoanalytic theory. Freud intelligently used the material he gathered to illustrate didactically his concepts of child sexuality, castration anxiety and the Oedipus complex.

However, Hans unexpectedly began to present phobic symptoms, transforming the research into treatment. Freud exercised the pioneering roles of *clinical supervisor* – he received the father's notes and discussed the contents with him – and of *family therapist* – he treated the father and son together and had already treated the mother individually, as noted. The father, while his main role was as a father, also took on the role of being supervised and the role of therapist. The work takes place in a positive transferential atmosphere in relation to Freud that can be observed in some comments that come from Hans. In a conversation in which his father asks Hans why he is afraid, Hans responds, "I don't know. But Professor Freud should know why. Don't you think he will know?" (p. 57). Returning to Freud's office, Hans comments to his father, "Does Professor Freud converse with God? It seems like he already knows everything beforehand" (p. 52).

The case takes place when Hans was from three to five years old. The period of "learning" relationship–separation, according to Bowlby, takes place, more or less, between six to nine months and five years of age. In effect, we shall observe that beside the sexual curiosity of the boy, as Freud points out, evidence of separation anxiety toward his mother, his father, and his home appears.

At four years and nine months of age, Hans awakes in tears saying to his mother, "When I was sleeping, I thought you had gone away and I was without a mother . . . imagine if I did not have a mother" (p. 34). These manifestations were not only directed toward his mother but also toward his father: "Imagine if you were to go away" (p. 34). Further, we see the following dialogue between father and son:

FATHER: "When you are alone, do you become anxious and come to talk with me?"

HANS: "When you are away, I become afraid that you will not come home."

FATHER: "And did I ever threaten to not return home?"

HANS: "Not you, but Mother did; Mother told me that she would not return."

FATHER: "She said that because you had been up to some mischief."

HANS: "Yes."

FATHER: "You become afraid that I will go away because you were naughty; for this reason you come close to me."

(Freud, 1976, p. 54).

The father always bases his comments on the Oedipal hypothesis of desire–guilt for paternal death. Without disagreeing, I would like to emphasize that either concomitantly or prior, there is a greater desire–fear than separation anxiety that is indistinct in relation to the father or mother. Hans goes through a phase in which he tries to "unmelt" himself from the matrix of identity (sociometry constituted by primary connections), but feels afraid. He tries to recognize himself as a person in the world (*recognition of I*) and to know other people (*recognition of You*). At this moment a third person emerges, offering him another relational possibility: to transform his vision of the world of two (symbiotic) to a broader world of three, which introduces his group insertion into the community. Passion for the third person is the anesthesia for the disconnection with the second person: "Father, you are so handsome! You are so fair" (p. 63). Hans goes through the process of forming the existential identity (elaboration of the relationship/separation complex), the sexual identity (he learns to be a man from his father) and the relational sexual identity (in sexual games with his friends).

Later, the boy begins to show fear in being far from home. At night he becomes frightened, cries and wishes to sleep in his parents' bedroom, which the father interprets as his son's desire to sleep alone with his mother. The mother decides to take Hans on a trip, "to be able to observe what torments him" (p. 35). Hans opposes the idea but in the end agrees. During the trip, Hans becomes frightened, referring to a horse that bites him. His father concludes that Hans suffers from a phobia of the streets, but the most coherent explanation would be to say that he presents a fear of leaving his house, because his real fear is to leave behind the security which that base, the matrix, represents.

Freud explains that Hans's sadness derives from a "certain intensification of his libido . . . because the object of such intensification was his mother, and perhaps his objective had been to sleep with her" (p. 36). Without repudiating this hypothesis, we can also consider that a night simply means the end of the day, and this alone represents a separation. Sleeping may mean the distancing of dear persons, a farewell to others and to oneself, a symbolic death. We must also remember to consider the separation which occurred when Hans was "exiled from his parents' room" (p. 138) after his sister was born. In the same sense, we can understand that when Hans insists on going into the bathroom with his mother he is not interested only in watching his mother go "lumf" (defecate) but is also desperate to maintain visual contact with her.

Hans's anxiety in relation to separation increases. He discovers the risks of loss in bizarre situations. Besides the phobic elements, obsessive elements present themselves in his attempts to control the threats to his psychological integrity. He appears to fear the sound of the toilet flushing: "Here (in Vienna), I am not afraid. In Lainz I am afraid when you pull the chain. And when I am in there and the water goes running down I am also afraid." As you can see, the fear is not only of the sound but also of the water that drains away (and that could take him with it). This manifestation is considered normal in small children. Still, he is afraid that if his mother leaves him alone in the bathroom he could drown, as he wishes would happen to his younger sister. From a young age, Hans had demonstrated a tendency toward intestinal constipation, which was corrected with nutritional guidance. In the period of the phobia, "the constipation returned somewhat frequently" (p. 65). It is a coherent symptom, if we take into consideration that the predominant experience of the patient is fear of losses and losing control – in this case, intestinal.

Hans goes through a phase in which he is working through the integration of partial/total, inside/outside, fantasy/reality, body/psyche; the symptoms which present themselves at five years of age are mere accidents leading to the construction of the adult personality. In this way, the characteristics of the intestinal functioning are no longer biological but biopsychological; in other words, they become a part of his *mode* of being, as we shall see later in "Roles and their modes (pp. 41–45).

The manifestations of anxiety (despair), anger (hate) and sadness (depression) referred to by Bowlby in the process of separation can be abundantly observed in this case. However, it is worth commenting on the hate that is associated, in Freud's report, with the desire for his father's death so that he can take possession of his mother, or when the hate is directed to the mother, charged with "obscure sadistic desires" (p. 136). From a relational point of view, anger, at first glance, can be considered a direct expression of abandonment. If this is valid, there are two types of anger present: one is direct, primary and dual, and the other is complex, competitive and triangular. Consequently, the guilt related to both angers will also be different. Of course, one can argue that in a situation of abandonment (dual), the "third" is always implicit and that the Oedipus complex (triangulation) is inborn. But perhaps this is a point in psychology where belief is worth more than clinical observation. Moreno believes that the psychoanalytic focus of the Oedipal drama is correct; he considers the Oedipal complex to be like an individual reaction. However, to represent the complete drama, an analysis of all the interactions in play would be necessary. The point of view of each involved in the relational network must be studied. In this way, we would have an Oedipal complex, a Laio complex and a Jocasta complex.

The relational focus of the "Little Hans Case" reveals a distinct philosophical position adapted from Freudian psychology. "Learning" relationship (life)/separation (death) is central to the relational approach since it forms the existential basis of human development; it precedes, in philosophical importance, the position which Freudian psychoanalysis gives to sexuality. This continues to be an important relational channel of the human being, but not the core of a psychological system. Castration anxiety, in turn, is derived from the "fear–anger–sadness" of separation. Finally, the Oedipal complex appears to be embodied in the process of triangulation, which coordinates the passage of the dual relationship (symbiosis and "corridor relationships") to the triangular relationship.

Fortunately, Hans improves: "His improvement has been constant. The radius of his circle of activities, with the front gate as center, becomes increasingly larger. He was even able to manage, which until now had been impossible, to run to the sidewalk on the other side of the street" (p. 63). This reminds us that the human being's course through life begins in the mother's womb, proceeds to her lap, follows to the floor, then to the backyard, to the block, through the neighborhood, to the city and to the world, yet never without missing the old "home". This is how it was with Hans: he grew up; he faced his parent's separation as an adolescent; later he left his home for the United States, where he became the scenic director of the Metropolitan Opera House in New York. But he would sometimes remember the period in his childhood that made him famous. He reappeared to "Herr Professor" in 1922, and to his daughter Anna Freud in 1970, telling her: "I am Little Hans."

We could not conclude these considerations without emphasizing the most psychodramatic moment of the account. Hans's father describes it in this manner: "For some time, Hans has pretended that he is a horse, in his room; he trots, he falls, kicks his feet about and whinnies. Once, he tied a bag to his face, similar to a horse's feeding bag. All of a sudden he ran up to me and bit me." The "psychodramatist" Freud comments on the strength of this dramatization: "In this sense, he accepts the interpretations with more determination than was possible with words, but naturally through a role reversal, in that the game unfolded following a fantasy full of desire. He was the horse and bit his father, and in this way identified with his father" (p. 61).

Global *I* and partial *I(s)*

As we saw in the "Little Hans Case", in order to comprehend the process of internalizing affective relationships in childhood, we must use the "partial/total" parameter. For example, from a concrete point of view, the "baby/mother's breast" relationship is partial, while the "child/mother" relationship is whole. Relationships, however, are internalized in a way so absolutely particular that they always represent partial acquisitions of the whole – firstly, because the relationship as a whole is perhaps more idealized than real, and, secondly, because the child is neurologically immature at this phase and his/her perceptive processes are rudimentary. The succession of repeated relational moments forms the process of internalization.

Relationships are internalized via scenes which have been experienced. These are to relationships like frames are to paintings. Scenes give the spatial–temporal reference and the affective color of the internalized relationships. Through a series of partial internalizations of relationships, internal partial $I(s)$ begin to sketch themselves. These begin with identification with both poles of the relationship. In this manner, in an internalized relationship A–B, the internal partial I will have characteristics of A, of B, and of A/B. If we imagine that the relationships are internalized as "good relationships" and "bad relationships", according to difficult relational experiences, we may conclude that both positive and negative partial $I(s)$ exist. In this sense, the child will internalize a constellation of mothers, where the good mother and the bad mother are only extremes of a process that encompasses positive and negative figures (with charges), to a varied degree. Such a constellation of "*negative $I(s)$*" could be responsible for the sensation of inner cruelty and the desire for self-punishment in certain obsessive personalities, for example.

The internal partial $I(s)$ and their constellations either come to the relational surface by way of role performance or they remain latent awaiting release. Formation of the internal partial $I(s)$ happens in the matrix of identity by exercising psychosomatic roles, imaginary (or fantasy) roles, and social roles. We will return to discuss these further ahead.

In this light, the psyche is comprised of a dynamic structure where the global I is formed by multiple partial $I(s)$ which sometimes group together in constellations, such as those of the *censor $I(s)$*, those of the *sado-masochistic $I(s)$*, etc. The internal partial $I(s)$ present a variable degree of relationship, which we may call *internal sociometry*. The individual relates, therefore, with groups of people (*I–you*, *I–they*, and *I–we*) and internally, with groups of internal $I(s)$ (*I–I*) – the internal and external group, and internal and external sociometry. Within this concept, however, the intrapsyche is an interrelation of the internal $I(s)$. It is worth noting, then, that the "intrapsychic" is "interpsychic" (interpersonal). Therefore, even when the psychotherapist dedicates him/herself to individual psychother-apy, it is really group psychotherapy because he/she is working with the internal group of the individual. The constellations of more active $I(s)$ form grooves that lead to the primary and secondary personality traits. Furthermore, from this perspective, narcissism can be understood as a state of the personality (*global I*) in which the partial internal $I(s)$ are polarized by a centripetal movement.[5]

Among the innumerable $I(s)$ which populate our psyche, we may add (inspired by Buber's "being and appearing"), the *apparent I* (who we appear to be or think we are) and the *real I* (who we are and struggle to recognize). The exaggerated development of the *apparent I* may give rise to the *false I*. Moreover, I include the *observer I* in this gallery, which neither applauds nor criticizes, but adequately captures who and how we are. Personal growth is directly connected to the development of the *observer I*; only through it can the psychotherapeutic process be successful. The *observer I* maintains the observation distance necessary ("distance and relation" from Martin Buber) to evaluate the partial internal $I(s)$ fairly.

---

5 Other ideas about this theme may be found in Chapter 4 'Personality Diagnosis and Identity Disorders'.

Dreams offer a didactic vision of the partial internal *I(s)*. These express themselves through oneiric (from Greek *oneiros*: dream) characters. The partial internal *I(s)* are the "actors" of oneiric theater. From this concept, a practical method in working with dreams is to encourage the patient to dramatize different oneiric characters. This way, the patient will not only be identifying with his/her internal *I(s)* but will also have a chance to psychodramatically "bring them into consciousness".

In order to evaluate some further aspects of relational psychology I will present another clinical case from psychoanalytic literature, the "Dora Case".

Relational focus of the Dora case

Freud's Dora case (1968, pp. 605–658), when considered within the relational focus, must take into account all of the relational possibilities by grouping Dora, her father, her mother, Mr K, Mrs K, and Freud, in all of the sociometric alternatives – the isolated member, the different dyads, trios, quartets, quintets, and the sextet, according to the forces of attraction, repulsion and neutrality. One should also take into account the form in which Dora internalized her primary relationships, her partial internal *I(s)* into *good I(s)* and *bad I(s)* in the matrix of identity. Dora was the "identified patient" (the first symptoms appeared at 8 years of age) from a saturated and pathological relational network.

The father (who Freud had previously treated for syphilis) and Mrs K were lovers, to the knowledge of Mr K, who benefited from this commercially. Mr K, in turn, had sexually harassed Dora since she was 14 years old. She reacted with fear and disgust. Her father, an accomplice, did not respond to Dora's pleas for help. Dora told her mother what was happening, "so that she would tell her husband that Mr. K dared to make sexual advances" (p. 610). Dora had a devoted friendship with Mrs K, which later became a deception ("unconscious homosexual link"). Apparently, the mother would watch all of this distantly. Dora's father and Mr K were "friends", despite, or perhaps due to, the fact that one was sleeping with the other's wife and the other was "flirting" with the adolescent daughter of the former. Freud gives his testimony and expresses his personal evaluation by considering the physical repugnance that Dora had for Mr K to be the fruit of sexual repression:

> Dora's repugnance, upon being kissed, surely did not depend on accidental circumstances which she would have remembered or mentioned. I had previously known Mr. K as someone who would accompany Dora's father once in a while to my office, and I knew that he was a man who was still young and attractive.

> (Freud, 1968, p. 612)

Freud did not consider that Dora could have been disgusted by the conspiratorial plot of the adults whom she attempted to denounce. He firmly maintained his classification "without hesitating, any person as hysterical where sexual excitement provokes disgust" (Freud, in Rodrigué, 1995, vol. 2, p. 47). Dora contests being considered a lying adolescent. Emilio Rodrigué (1995, vol. 2, p. 48) refers to this point: "Continuing with this task of 'supervising' Freud, the flood of interpretations is alarming. His refusal to consider Dora's doubts as anything beyond mere resistance is also impressive." Further, Rodrigué refers to Freud's later recognition of his error, saying that he was not able to "manage" the transference. A clinical error that, incidentally, did not impede the scientific/literary success of the case.

Dora hoped for validation by capturing her familiar reality. She had hopes that the entrance of the sixth element, Freud, could modify the previous system and relieve her from the condition of identified patient. There was, in addition to Dora's symptoms, a relational neurosis. However, she received interpretations that, despite being theoretically correct, invalidated her in her social network. What was important to Freud was the sexual attraction that Dora denied and not her existential experience within her social atom. For this reason, Dora understandably refused to continue treatment, retaliating against the family and doctor who did not understand her.

Freud, in his obsession for the "unconscious (intrapsychic) truth", becomes blind to the "relational (interpersonal) truth". Within the first condition, the "other" is secondary or does not exist and the perspective of the relationship is lost – the "other" is always internalized only. This attitude generates a psychotherapeutic position where the privilege is given to only one of the "truths". On the other hand, an attitude that emphasizes only the external relational "truth", to the detriment of the internal "truth", would also be partial. I think that it is possible to conciliate the two "truths" in a relational psychology that includes the *I–I* relationship (internal truth) and the *I–you* (external truth). This attitude is consistent with new scientific paradigms, which recognize that all theories are limited. Science cannot obtain a definitive comprehension of reality, and scientists always deal with approximate descriptions of such reality. For this reason, the reader who is passionate about an author should remember that the truth is not *only* but *also* what he/she is reading.

These comments, by the way, about the "Dora case" reveal that there are other angles to be explored by studying the relational dynamic of this diabolic quintet, or sextet – without missing the pun: sex-tet, given the number and the intensity of the sexual currents involved. In the first place, as previously mentioned, Dora cannot be identified as the only "sick person" in the saturated relational network. In the second place, our attention is called to the fact that, although there is an "unconscious truth" to be discovered, there is also a "conscious truth" to be confronted. Finally, for an adolescent of 17 years of age, even without considering aspects of her personality, to know that her father is the lover of a woman she had admired and who she had modeled as a woman (as the saying goes: "when I grow up I want to be just like him/her"); and to realize that the oldest man whom she had liked, the "uncle", was not a hero but a conspirator with hidden interests involved in a maddening farce that the adults, including Freud, enacted around her; and to further have a weak mother who was not able to protect her ("housewife psychosis"[6]), were already more than enough reasons to have had many hysterical fits and demonstrate disgust toward anyone.

In outlining these ideas, I cannot help fantasizing about the participants gathered with Dr Freud in his office, Freud enacting his first family group psychotherapy session. It must have been a grandiose premiere.

The universal relational dimension of man

In this internal (intra) and external (inter) relational dynamic, an "activity", which we may very well call "energy", is implicit if we restrict ourselves to the concepts of flow, flotation, vibration, rhythm, synchronism and resonance.[7] Just as, according to Freud, the libido seeks pleasure, in this concept the "energy" seeks relationships, enabling one to speak of a relational "instinct" (or "impulse"). This comes from the supposition that in the universe everything is energy and everything is a relationship. As Einstein taught us, matter is energy in a condensed state, and energy is matter in a radiant state. Man, however, is both matter and energy, and relates to other similar and dissimilar matters and energies. The human being possesses a variable chemical–electromagnetic energy depending on his/her feelings, thoughts, sensations, and his/her state of sickness–health; this can be measured, at least in part, by medical equipment (electroencephalograph, cerebral mapping, electromyography, magnetic resonance, etc.).

In one sense, the concept of the "conscious–unconscious" is connected to the concept of energy. Metaphorically, we can understand this by comparing light to the conscience. Mental phenomena can be lighter or darker, depending on the light (conscience) that shines upon them. In this comparison we have two extremes, one very dark and one very light, with a zone of light-to-dark in between. The lighter dark corresponds to the pre-conscious (and the pre-unconscious). The dark corresponds to the unconscious and the very dark to the transpersonal unconscious, like Jung's collective unconscious.

---

6 Expression from Rodrigué (1995, vol. 2, p. 42) about Freud's reference to the "symptoms of this disinterested and common nosologic entity: disinterest in one's children, obsession for cleanliness, total lack of insight for the nature of one's disease, coldness".

7 I use some points from Capra (1988).

The light zone refers to the conscious and the very light to the supra-conscious. The supra-conscious occupies the states of consciousness experienced in special moments, outside the normal sphere – "peak experiences" – as in the *encounter* (from Moreno and Buber). The supra-conscious is also present in varying degrees during meditative states (non-thinking), which are achieved by deliberately focusing attention on oneself.[8]

If the universe is understood to be the relationship of all its elements, we have to search for man's position in this relational network. What is his position in time and space? Nicoll (1979) considers man to be composed of an essence and a personality. The human being is born with an essence, corresponding to the inner human microcosm. The microcosm has the same "substance" or "energy" as the macrocosm. For this reason, the image of God is common "within" (microcosm) man, or, "above" (macrocosm) him, in the sky. Thus, man is connected to the universe (ray of creation) through his essence, and connected to Earth through his personality. Personality formation originates from the psychological and social development of the human being and could be likened to a "wrapping" of the essence, this being the object of traditional psychological studies. We have, then, two perspectives of the human being: a vertical one, through the essence (cosmos), and a horizontal one, through the personality (Earth). Man lives at the intersection of these two lines.

These points permit us to understand the encounter (from Buber and Moreno) as an impact that dissolves the personalities involved (loss of momentary identity), promoting contact of the essences and liberation of energy ("divine sparks" from Moreno). They also permit us to clarify the cosmic component of the human being that Moreno noted so many times in his work.

The cosmic dimension of man can be visualized as his "hierarchical" relational position in the universe. Man is part of the organic material of planet Earth, which has a satellite (moon), and together with the other planets revolves around the sun, forming a large astronomic relational system called the galaxy (Milky Way). This, in turn, belongs to a group of infinite galaxies, which comprise the universe or the absolute. Man is part of this whole (system); therefore, he influences it and is influenced by it.

Roles and their modes[9]

Moreno's role theory and the psychoanalytic concept of erogenous zones and phases can be linked. I believe that this results in creative subsidies to

---

8 For more detailed information, see Chapter 6.
9 I am inspired by Erik Erikson (1976), who offers a concept of erogenous zones in accordance with their "modes and modalities" of action.

the study of the relational phenomenon. To make this connection, we must dedicate some consideration to the period of human development in which these events happen.

Psychoanalytic theory states that the libido is organized according to the priority of erogenous zones, according to the predominance of "object relationship" modalities. For example, some mucous membrane zones are prevalent in the relationship of the baby with his/her environment. This organization happens in the pre-genital phases – oral, anal, and phallic – that precede the initiation of the genital phase. This developmental step is characterized by functions such as sucking, biting, excreting, retaining, penetrating, looking, smelling, hearing, etc. The child begins to devise modes of being, starting from an imaginative elaboration of sensorial perceptions, which originate from the body functions. In this way, the experience of the organic *modes* corresponds to the future psychological *modes* of the individual.

Moreno studies the development of roles in the *matrix of identity*. This development begins with psychosomatic (biological) roles, then passes to imaginary (psychological) roles, and finally reaches social roles, through which connections with the counter-roles of other people are established. Psychosomatic roles and imaginary roles constitute the basic internal structure of the social roles through which the individual will relate in adult life.

To understand the origin of psychosomatic roles, we must use the Morenian concept of the "zone". The zone is comprised of the

> group of self-elements and foreign elements, acting and present, that intervene in the exercise of an indispensable function. The zone involves, therefore, the organic elements and extra-organic elements that establish solid ties between the individual and his environment. These ties are increasingly reinforced as the zone goes into action – that is to say, when all of its components coincide in focus. It is through this repeated and prolonged contact that the psychosomatic roles acquire their total development and maturity and lay the bases for the later development of social and dramatic roles.
>
> (Rojas-Bermudez, 1975, p. 53)

The psychopathological study of disorders connected to the zone should, consequently, take into consideration all of the elements which are present in the system at hand. The zone, therefore, does not happen "in" the baby but in the relationship established between the baby and his/her *matrix of identity*. The zone represents the "energetic corridor" made up of the baby, the mother, and all of the biological, psychological, and cultural circumstances inherent to both. The zone is active when energy flows through this "corridor" or relational channel. This movement causes the roles involved in the act to emerge, establishing a connection and corresponding relationship. The zone becomes subjacent, therefore, to all relational phenomena in the child as well as the adult. In any act, be it nursing for the child or sex for the adult, both individual and reciprocal "warming up" takes place, becoming the focus, which triggers the movement of the zone. This, in turn, fosters the appearance of the respective roles and counter-roles, literally configuring the link and the act.

Roles present two dimensions because they are structured by both collective and individual components. They are collective in that they contain cultural elements, which belong to the individual ("social unit of conduct" from Moreno). The components are individual in respect to the individual's personal history. For example, the role of a doctor contains elements that are common to the micro and macro society in which he/she belongs, and particular elements in relation to a specific doctor. In other words, the individual brings the connotation of his/her person to the performance of social roles in a community. There are, for example, doctors who are receptive, attentive, conservative, daring, innovative, direct, aggressive, etc.

To summarize, zones create individual modes of being, or better, modes of establishing relationships. This devising of relational personality characteristics begins with the imaginative elaboration of how the body functions are experienced and how they serve as a relational instrument for the child in his/her environment. This result is expressed through exercising roles. Every role contains historic registers within the imaginative elaboration of the oral, anal, and phallic phases, or from the roles of ingestor, defecator and urinator, and from all the other psychosomatic roles, such as the roles of breather, sleeper, dreamer, watcher, smeller, listener, etc.

In this stage of development, the child establishes limits between inside/outside, good/bad, partial/whole, and fantasy/reality. The "movement" ("course") between one state and another is included in this discriminatory process. This movement connects, in both directions, the "inside" and the "outside", or, the body's "entrance" and the "exit". This movement can be observed at two moments:

- in the relationship with oneself ("recognition of I" from Moreno's matrix of identity), *what and how something enters in me, and what and how something exits me,* and
- in the relationship with the "other" ("recognition of you" from Moreno's matrix of identity), *what and how I can put something in the other, and what and how I can protect something inside of me from the other.*

If we take into consideration the "law of two" or the "law of the complement" from nature (cold/hot, day/night, dry/humid, etc.), we must consider three things: what enters, what exits, and *what enters and exits*, as part of any single relational process. Further, we should consider *how* this process happens, in that the inside–outside–inside movement can occur in different ways. It could be fast or slow, active or passive, continuous or discontinuous, affectionate or aggressive, and so on. In this sense, taking into consideration both *what* and *how*, the process as a whole begins to be inscribed in the child's memory (conscious–unconscious) and is part of the *mode* of how he/she will act out his/her roles in adult life. In other words, the social roles of this person will follow a performance *modality* of all the social roles. *Mode* is understood as a personal characteristic that becomes visible in the performance of all social roles. For instance, an adult man will allow a common aspect, a "trademark" (a mode) to become visible in all his social roles – as husband, father, boss, coworker, or athlete – devised during the formation of his psychosomatic roles and imagination. As systemic theory states that the elements of the whole also exist in the partial, we may say that the careful study of any role reveals the main characteristics of the personality as a whole.

To better describe this period of human development we need to find denominations that preserve the aspect of *how* this process happens. I propose that we call them:

1   The incorporative-eliminatory phase.
2   The intrusive-receptive phase.

The incorporative-eliminatory phase (excretory, expulsive) is connected to the "recognition of *I*", the parameter being the physical–psychological conscience of everything that enters and exits the individual. In this sense, the human being not only eats through the mouth, but incorporates through the mouth, eyes, nose, ears and touch; in other words, through his/her whole being. There are three forms of nourishment essential to man: food (digestive nourishment), oxygen (respiratory nourishment) and impressions (sensorial nourishment). The eliminatory (excretory) process occurs in the same way, not only through the physical excretion of feces and urine but also through the symbolic representation of these physiological functions. This includes everything leaving the individual, whether acts, thoughts or emotions.

From the relational point of view, then, the incorporative-eliminatory phase incorporates the oral and anal phases of psychoanalytic theory and the roles of ingestor, defecator and urinator – the "Nucleus of *I*" theory from Rojas-Bermudez (1975).

In the second phase, the intrusive-receptive phase, linked to the "recognition of you", the parameter is everything that enters our physical–psychic border, how it is "made to enter", as well as everything that we "make enter" the border of another. The connotation of to penetrate and to be penetrated gains a broad relational context. The sexual aspect is literally contained within the intrusive-receptive aspect. The intrusive-receptive phase embodies, within a relational perspective, the phallic phases of psychoanalytic theory and, in part, the role of the urinator from Rojas-Bermudez.

This approach to the *role and its modes* highlights the manner in which the formation process happens. The affective "atmosphere" experienced by the child in the development of his/her roles must be taken into account. This atmosphere reflects different nuances according to the circumstances of development. Broadly, the incorporative part of the incorporative-eliminatory zone is responsible, to different degrees, for "learning", *receive/take/yank (steal)*, and its opposite, *refuse/reject/repudiate (disgust)* – different modes of experiencing what and how something crosses one's borders. The eliminatory part of the incorporative-eliminatory zone is in charge of "learning" the process of *give (release)/toss/throw/(expel)* and the opposite, *conserve (save)/retain/imprison* – different modes of experiencing what and how something exits.

In the same way, the *intrusion-reception* phase generates different role modalities according to its mode of action. The intrusive zone is responsible for the modes of *enter (fulfill)/penetrate (explore)/invade (conquer)* – different modes of crossing the limits of the other. The receptive zone embodies the modes of *protect/keep/hide* – different modes of receiving the other within us.

Role modes can be studied not only through the range of intensity of their characteristics but also through the level of activity–passivity in their performance. The analysis of human attitudes and behaviors, expressed through the performance of roles, becomes enriched if we consider the characteristics according to the circumstances of the relationships in which they are established. In this manner, the concept of "healthy/pathological" has much more to do with the flexibility and appropriateness of a role in its link (with its counter-role) than with an arbitrary analysis of its value. Different degrees of a mode (for example, *enter/penetrate/invade* or *protect/keep/hide*) may be appropriate or not, depending on the relational balance that exists in the particular link. What is inappropriate in the "invasive" mode of a thief is appropriate for the soldier who "penetrates" enemy territory. Likewise, while the act of sexually "invading" a woman without consent and impregnating her is aggressive, it is also aggressive for a woman sexually to betray a man and "hide" (*yank/rob*) her intention to become pregnant.

Accordingly, I believe that an endless series of combinations and inter-actions within the role modes and their links is opened.

Physical, psychological and energetic body[10]

The aspect of child development approached in the previous section plays a part in identity formation. The identity passes through a physical–psychological definition of the individual's corporeal limits. Thus, we may speak of a "zonal identity", to the extent that a child defines, through action and repetition, a "corporeal area" and a "relational area" with his/her environment ("corridor or relational channel"). Thus, the oral zone defines not only the mouth area but also all of the anatomic-physiological structures involving the mouth area and the maternal breast, and, mainly, the energy (biological, psychological, and cultural) involved in this relational channel. For example, after the oral zone, there is the action of the anal zone and the concretization of the consciousness of the mouth–anus segment (digestive track), a "segmentary identity". Beginning with the segmentary identities, we arrive at a "total identity" of the whole body. From the relational point of view, the whole corporeal identity also signifies a consciousness of the environment and the inherent relationships to the matrix of identity (capacity for role reversal). From a philosophic point of view, however, nobody arrives at a "complete" identity, perfect knowledge of him/herself and of others; in other words, a god.

Our bodies are limited by who we are and who we imagine ourselves to be. There are physical and psychological limits of the body that are compared to their respective imaginative representation (self-image). It is worth noting, therefore, that the physical body (real) is perhaps more credibly revealed by way of the *other*'s eye than by our own, which is always under the influence of the psychological (symbolic) body. These are the origins of the concepts of *physical body* and *psychological* (symbolic) *body*. The *energetic body* is the result of the (psychic–corporeal) interaction between them. This interaction can occur with more or less spontaneous fluency. The existence of conflicts results in tension and communicational "noise", altering the spontaneous physical–corporeal fluency between the bodies. The state of ideal health (bio-psychic-social) requires a "silent", fluent, and spontaneous energetic body, the fruit of "noiseless" communication between the physical and psychological bodies. On the other hand, one may have a sick physical body, but with good spontaneous fluency in relation to the psychological body, which results in an energetic, relatively balanced body, despite the existence of physical sickness. The same sickness, therefore, can present various evolutions according to the interaction between the physical and the psychological bodies; that is, in accordance with the present energetic body.

10 Other comments about this theme may be found in Chapter 7.

Laing and relational psychology

In concluding this review of the theories which have had an influence on me, I could not forget Ronald Laing. In the 1970s I "subversively" referred his readings to my medical residents, since he was a *persona non grata* among the heads of psychiatry at that time. The most important author of the anti-psychiatry movement, despite his romantic and mystic exuberance, he left a consistent foundation for relational psychology. His phenomenological–existential foundations approximate those of Buber and Moreno, although he had probably not read Moreno.[11] While Laing made many contributions, more than anything else he left a relational philosophy. Rather than stating his concepts, perhaps the best way to transmit his philosophy would be to recount an occurrence that took place when he was in São Paulo in 1978. During the supervision of psychiatrists and psychoanalysts, Laing related the case of a schizophrenic patient who so adamantly refused to bathe he had reached the point of smelling quite strongly. At the same time, the young man complained of his difficulty in approaching women. At this point Laing interrupted his story, asking what the appropriate technical attitude was for the situation. A flood of psychodynamic hypotheses were suggested, each cleverer than the last. The most accepted theory, however, was that the patient did not bathe to avoid realizing his incestuous desires. Women rejected him for smelling badly, which saved him from Oedipal concretization. After many interpretations, Laing retorted that perhaps water represented amniotic fluid to this man; when wet, the patient would feel as if he were within the uterus and, therefore, in total Oedipal "sin". The group was overwhelmed by the shrewdness of the grand master! When the compliments came to an end, Laing added: "I told him that his smell was unpleasant and that it was unpleasant to be with him. Despite my interest in his treatment, if he did not come to the following session clean, I would no longer treat him."

He paused and then completed the story: "In the next session, as well as those following, he arrived freshly bathed!"

Conclusion

I hope to have synthesized the main theories that have influenced my conceptions about personality development. These influences can be understood under the guidance of a relational psychology. In addition to some technical proposals that are translated in Relationship Psychotherapy and in Internal Psychodrama (techniques which I have developed), these concepts comprise my attempt to contribute to contemporary psychodrama.

---

11 See Fonseca (1977). El psicodrama y la psiquiatria: Moreno y la anti-psiquiatri (Psycho-drama and psychiatry: Moreno and anti-psychiatry). *Momento*, 3, 4–5: 39–45.

Once again, the image of the young man returns from the beginning of this text. His question about my line of psychotherapeutic work inspired this long response. If he could read this, he would ask further questions, because as Moreno says (1977) in his motto: "More important than science is its result; one answer provokes a hundred questions . . ."

References

Anzieu, D. (1961). *El Psicodrama analítico en el niño (Analytic psychodrama in children)*. Buenos Aires: Paidós. (Original edition: *Le psychodrame analytique chez l'enfant*. Paris: Presses Universitaires de France, 1956.)

Bowlby, J. (1982). *Formação e rompimento dos laços afetivos*. São Paulo: Martins Fontes. (Original edition: *The making and breaking of affectional bonds*. London: Tavistock Publications, 1979.)

Buber, M. (1957). Distance and relation. *Psychiatry*, 20, 2: 97–104.

Capra, F. (1988). *O ponto de mutação*. Cultrix: São Paulo. (Original edition: *The turning point*. New York/London: Simon and Schuster/Wildwood House, 1982.)

Erikson, E. (1976) *Infância e sociedade*. Rio de Janeiro: Zahar. (Original edition: *Childhood and society*. New York: W. W. Norton & Company, Inc., 1963.)

Fairbairn, W. R. (1975). *Estudio psicanalítico de la personalidad*. Buenos Aires: Hormé. (Original edition: *Psychoanalytic studies of the personality*. London: Tavistock Publications, 1952.)

Figueiredo, C. (1949). *Dicionário da líqua portuguesa (Portuguese Language Dictionary)*. Lisboa/Rio de Janeiro: Bertrand-Jackson.

Fonseca, J. (1977). El psicodrama y la psiquiatria: Moreno y la anti-psiquiatri (Psychodrama and psychiatry: Moreno and anti-psychiatry). *Momento*, 3, 4–5: 39–45.

Fonseca, J. (1980). *Psicodrama da loucura (Psychodrama of madness)*. São Paulo: Ágora.

Fonseca, J. (1989). Psicologia do adoecer (The psychology of becoming ill). Presented at the Brazilian Congress of Obstetrics, São Paulo.

Fonseca, J. (1994). O doente, a doença e o corpo. Visão através do psicodrama interno (The patient, the illness and the body. A vision through internal psychodrama). *Revista Brasileira de Psicodrama*, 2, I: 41–48.

Fonseca, J. (1995). Diagnóstico da personalidade e distúrbios de identidade (Personality diagnosis and indentity disorders). *Revista Brasileira de Psicodrama*, 3, I: 21–29.

Fonseca, J. (1996a). Ainda sobre a matriz de identidade (More on the matrix of identity). *Revista Brasileira de Psicodrama*, 4, II: 21–34.

Fonseca, J. (1996b). Psicodrama interno (Internal psychodrama). *Leituras*, 16: 1–6.

Freud, S. (1967). *Psicologia de las masas (Psychology of the masses)*. Obras Completas, I. Madrid: Editorial Biblioteca Nueva.

Freud, S. (1968). *Analisis fragmentario de una histeria (Dora's case)*. Obras Completas, II, pp. 605–658. Madrid: Editorial Biblioteca Nueva. (English edition: *Fragment of an analysis of a case of hysteria*. Complete Psychological Works of Sigmund Freud, vol. VII, pp. 51–52. London: Hogarth Press, 1905.)

Freud, S. (1976). *Análise de uma fobia em um menino de cinco anos (The case of little*

Hans). Edição Standard Brasileira das Obras Psicológicas Completas de Sigmund Freud, vol. X, pp. 15–154. Rio de Janeiro: Imago. (English edition: *Analysis of a phobia in a five-year-old boy.* Standard Edition, vol. 10, 1909.)

Garcia-Roza, L. A. (1993). *Freud e o inconsciente (Freud and the unconscious).* Rio de Janeiro: Zahar.

Gay, P. (1989). *Freud, uma vida para nosso tempo.* São Paulo: Companhia das Letras. (Original edition: *Freud, a life for our time.* New York/London: Norton, 1988.)

Holmes, P. (1996). *A exteriorização do mundo interior – o psicodrama e a teoria das relações objetais.* São Paulo: Ágora. (Original edition: *The inner world outside: object relations theory and psychodrama.* London: Routledge, 1992.)

Jung, C. G. (1995). Psicogênese das doenças mentais (Prefácio) (The psychogenes of mental illness). In: N. S. Vargas, Psicoterapia de casais: uma visão simbólica, arquetípica da conjugalidade (Couples psychotherapy: a symbolic, archetypical view of conjugality). Doctoral thesis presented at the School of Medicine at the University of São Paulo.

Lebovici, S., Diatkine, R. and Kestemberg, E. (1958). *Bilan de dixans de thérapeutique par le psychodrame chez l'enfant et l'adolescent.* Paris: Psychiatrie de L'enfant.

Mannoni, O. (1995) Ficções freudianas (Freudian fictions). In: E. Rodrigué, *Sigmund Freud: o século da psicanálise 1895–1995 (Sigmund Freud: the century of psychoanalysis 1895–1995)*, vol. 2, p. 48. São Paulo: Escuta.

Martinez Bouquet, C., Moccio, F. and Pavlovsky, E. (1971). *Psicodrama: cuando y por qué dramatizar (Psychodrama: When and why to dramatize).* Buenos Aires: Proteo.

Montoro, G. F. (1994). Contribuições da teoria do apego à terapia familiar (Contributions of attachment theory to family therapy). In: T. Castilho, *Temas em terapia familiar (Themes in family therapy)*, pp. 40–77. São Paulo: Plexus.

Moreno, J. L. (1977). *Psychodrama – First Volume* (5th edn). New York: Beacon House, Inc.

Naffah Neto, A. (1995). Papel imaginário (Imaginary role). In: C. M. Menegazzo, M. M. Zuretti and M. A. Tomasini, *Dicionário de psicodrama e sociodrama (The dictionary of psychodrama and sociodrama)*, p. 151. São Paulo: Ágora.

Nicoll, M. (1979). *Comentários psicológicos sobre las enseñanzas de Gurdjieff y Ouspensky.* Buenos Aires: Kier. (Original edition: *Psychological commentaries on the teaching of Gurdjieff and Ouspensky.* London: Vincent Stuart Publishers, 1952.)

Perazzo, S. (1995). Papel de fantasia (The role of fantasy). In: C. M. Menegazzo, M. M. Zuretti and M. A. Tomasini, *Dicionário de psicodrama e sociodrama (The dictionary of psychodrama and sociodrama)*, p. 149. São Paulo: Ágora.

Rodrigué, E. (1995). *Sigmund Freud: o século da psicanálise 1895–1995 (Sigmund Freud: the century of psychoanalysis 1895–1995).* São Paulo: Escuta.

Rojas-Bermudez, J. G. (1975). *Que és el psicodrama (What is psychodrama).* Buenos Aires: Genitor.

Schützenberger, A. A. and Weil, P. (1977). *Psicodrama triádico: Uma síntese entre Freud, Moreno, Kurt Lewin e outros (Triadic psychodrama: A synthesis among Freud, Moreno, Kurt Lewin and others).* Belo Horizonte: Interlivros.

Vargas, N. S. (1995). *Psicoterapia de casais: uma visão simbólica, arquetípica da conjugalidade (Couples psychotherapy: a symbolic, archetypical view of conjugality).* Doctoral thesis presented to the School of Medicine at the University of São Paulo.

Chapter 3

The psychology of becoming ill

The role of the caretaker*

From the time we are children we experience pain and infirmity. Childhood illnesses make up our first experiences in the role of the sick person. The counterpart, the ill person's caretaker, and the bonds that result from it, originate, therefore, within familiar bounds. Upon becoming ill, the child is cared for by adults who comprise his/her relational network of social insertion, the *matrix of identity* (Moreno, 1977). This internalized experience forms the basic structure of the roles of sick person and caretaker in the future adult. As most human beings die of some disease, the health/illness dyad is a constant from the beginning to the end of life.

The role of professional caretaker (which includes doctor, psychologist, social worker, and physical therapist – in short, medical professionals in general) originates from the personal experiences of frailty in childhood. To a certain extent, the role of professional caretaker contains within it prior experiences of being ill and of having been cared for. In this text, I emphasize the study of the roles and the patient–caretaker bond, but the considerations that follow could easily be transposed to the student–caretaker dyad.

Roles: relational structures

Roles represent the fundamental connections of the human relationship. The roles of sick person and caretaker form the foundation of the doctor/patient and psychologist/patient relationships, among others of this type. The roles of sick person and caregiver contain both individual and collective aspects. The way in which a person becomes ill reflects his historical-psychological profile and the cultural context in which he grew up. Moreno observes that social roles carried out in adulthood, such as the role of the sick person, contain the structural imprints of the psychosomatic and psychological roles carried out in childhood. Psychosomatic roles represent

---

* Text based on a presentation given at the Brazilian Congress on Obstetrics and Gynecology, São Paulo, 1989.

the way in which the child establishes his first relationship in the *matrix of identity* (the role of ingestor, urinator, defecator, sleeper, breather, etc.). Psychological roles represent the imaginary or fantasy experiences that occur during neuropsychological development. In this way, the social role of the ill person contains all the psychosociological registers of the experiences of becoming ill during childhood.

Tele–transference system

All relationships are involved in the *tele–transference system*. *Tele* refers to the mutually correct perception, apprehension or caption of the relationship experience between two or more people. *Transference*, on the other hand, is found in relationships where at least one of the members presents a perception, apprehension or caption which is distorted from the other or others. This happens when this member projects his/her internal world onto the other(s), the object(s) of this emotional polarization. There may be, therefore, one-way relational transference: from A to B or from B to A; or two-way transference: from A to B and from B to A. Although, from a theoretical point of view, relationships are either *telic* or transferential, from a practical point of view it may be more coherent to state that relationships are mixed (tele–transferential), oscillating continually between the two poles. Thus, depending on the moment, we have relationships which are either more *telic* or more transferential.

Relationships lean to the transferential pole when there is an increase in anxiety in the situation (locus). In crisis situations, there is a predisposition toward transferential reactions. For example, one individual may catch a cold yet continues life as usual. Another, supposedly with the same cold, takes medication and goes to work. Yet another loads up on medicines, stays in bed and seeks maternal caretaking from his/her spouse. These are three reactions with different levels of tele–transference which solicit complementary responses, equally tele–transferential. The third subject presents regressive responses, reacting along infantile behavioral lines. It is important to clarify that everyone presents transferential reactions which aren't, in and of themselves, synonymous with illness. The pathological aspect of transference reveals itself in its intensity, frequency, or continued appearance in an individual's different social roles.

If we take the study of human relationships to the scope of the physician–patient relationship, we will have a whole world to analyze. When seeking out a doctor, the patient is in a state of anxiety, which, as mentioned, is an invitation for the appearance of transferential reactions. The human being behind the role of doctor reacts to the transferential solicitations of this patient based on his/her personality and personal history. Counter-transferential relationships are, therefore, quite possible. The tele–transferential system (which includes counter-tele–transference) is the psychological substrate of the doctor–patient relationship in all medical specialties. In psychotherapies, the tele–transferential system is also a basic relational structure. Some psychotherapies favor working with the established patient–psychotherapist relationship (here and now); others, though they don't disregard this, focus on the issues of the patient's life outside the therapeutic context (there and then). But the patient–therapist relationship always underlies any other issue worked on in the psychotherapy session.

The ability to deal with relationships (tele–transference system) comes from the cradle, from the *matrix of identity*.[1] It is developed through practice in life and can be perfected with professional training groups (*role-playing*). The genuine talent for managing relationships (*interpersonal intelligence*) allied with, obviously, theoretical knowledge and a mastery of the techniques of his/her specialty, defines a great part of a doctor's or therapist's success.

The tele-transferential system covers not only person–person relationships but also person–object relationships. Thus, we can include the relationships of patients and doctors with institutions that provide medical services (in other words, the patient–institution and doctor–institution relationships) in this study. Such institutions receive tele–transferential emotional loads as much from patients as from doctors and medical professionals in general. Hospitals and emergency rooms receive, in addition to justified criticisms from a social–political–administrative point of view, attacks originating from personal frustrations and delusions: the loss of loved ones, feared diagnoses, physical consequences, etc. In analyzing the institutional doctor–patient relationship, this variable must be taken into account, as it is very different from the relationship established in a private doctor's office with no intermediary connections. When the patient utilizes a medical plan, even if the consultation or procedure takes place in a private clinic, the doctor–patient relationship is influenced by their respective feelings toward the institution and the therapeutic result may be altered as a consequence. In this way, the institution mediates the doctor–patient relationship according to the design shown in the diagram.

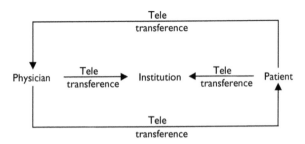

---

1 The *matrix of identity* is the source of the genetic, psychological, social and cosmic influences of the individual, according to Moreno (1977).

Relationship/separation: three basic psychodynamic positions

Moreno (1974) summarizes the development of the *matrix of identity* in three stages: (1) *the identity stage*, of *I* with *you*, of the subject with surrounding objects; (2) *the recognition of I* stage, of one's singularity as a person; and (3) *the recognition of you* stage, the recognition of others. Detailed observation of these psychological development phases reveals important points for the study of human psychosocial dynamics. There are three basic psychodynamic positions between the initial stage of total identity in relation to the surrounding environment and the *recognition of I* and *recognition of you* stages. These coordinate the psychodynamic understanding of the origin of the adult's *social role of the sick person* and the psycho(patho)logical nuances of falling ill. The basic psychodynamic positions organize the *learning to relate* and *learning to separate*, which, in truth, comprise two poles of the same process: relationship–separation. These positions form the foundation for the way in which the future adult establishes relationships (separations) with himself and others.

The first psychodynamic position refers to the learning of relationship–separation in itself. The second, related in another way to relationship–separation, is the formation of the individual's sense of self-worth, the conscious–unconscious understanding of the value the person attributes to himself (self-esteem) and of the value he/she is awarded in his social environment (esteem). The third basic psychodynamic position relates to the qualitative transformation of a two-person relationship to a triangular one and to the separation that the *intercessor* thus fosters within the prior unity.

The explanation of these basic psychodynamic positions will be presented in a didactic sequence, not necessarily following chronological order. In truth, the positions remain active throughout one's lifetime, always subject to reworking through existential experience or psychotherapy.

Relationship/separation

The first position coordinates the "learning" of being together and being alone. The pair of opposites (nature's "law of twos") relative to relationship–separation is always present in human life: sperm and ovum, separated and united (forming the zygote), pregnancy and birth, maternal caregiving or the lack of it, life–death, etc. As John Bowlby states (1981), the basic period of learning relationship–separation is from birth to approximately five or six years of age. In this phase, the basic relationship structures of loving and being loved, of loving and being rejected, and of rejecting are internalized. A child is first connected to surrounding human beings in a generic way, accepting caretaking indiscriminately. With neuropsychological maturation, the child begins to connect preferentially (primary sociometry), acquiring the capacity to choose people. In our culture, the mother is the child's primordial choice, but it is not uncommon for a grandmother, nanny, or the father to be the first choice. In any case, observation of the child's small relational world reveals the existence of preferential choices and a gradation among them. The child doesn't necessarily elect the person who provides the technically best maternal caretaking, but chooses someone with whom he/she feels closer and inspires the most trust ("holding" by Winnicott, 1978). When attachment develops, a child will prefer his/her inexperienced mother to a highly qualified nurse. Likewise, adults also choose friends, sexual partners, spouses, doctors, etc. according to varying criteria. For example, when a patient has references for several competent medical professionals, he will make a human choice, preferring the one who inspires more trust.

Consider the separation pole. A child exhibits a series of emotional reactions whenever his/her favored person threatens to remove or does remove him/herself. The first reaction, in the face of imminent loss, is anxiety. The second is anger for having been abandoned. In the third stage comes sadness from living with the loss. In the fourth and last stage, the process is resolved – within a period of time the child becomes well again, peacefully relating with the caretaker of the moment. These phases repeat themselves innumerable times throughout both childhood and adulthood. Additionally, the caretakers exhibit an affective counterpart (response) in relation to the child's emotional manifestations, which generates a relational network, a micro-social atom of attractions, neutralities and rejections – the child's primary sociometry in his *matrix of identity*.

Due to the suffering inherent in separating, the child develops psychological techniques for diminishing or avoiding the pain. This organized structure of avoiding suffering is given the name *the shock-absorber process* or *defense formation*. The *shock absorbers* or *defenses* are incorporated in the child's way of behaving, becoming a part of his personality as well. For example, in order to avoid the suffering that comes from loss, the child may react with indifference, a kind of affective anesthesia, as if he/she felt little or nothing (schizoid defense). Other diminishing techniques are known as obsessive, hysterical, phobic, paranoid, etc. defenses. In short, the *marks* of the different phases of separation (anxiety, anger/hatred, sadness/depression) added to the *marks* from defenses form grooves in the developing personality, becoming the primary and secondary personality traits. This primary psychological structure serves as the basis for all the processes of separation and loss in the future adult.

When ill, a person feels the threat of losing life. He/she fears losing relationships with others and with him/herself; he/she dreads the loneliness of death. And, just like a child facing imminent abandonment by his/her mother, he/she reacts with anxiety, anger and sadness, activating his/her shock absorbers or defenses. The medical professional is the first shield against which these expressions of alarm are thrown. It should be remembered that, in addition to the patient's reactions, there are also those of his/her family, anxious about the possibility of losing the patient. Doctors and medical workers know very well of patients and relatives who develop an anxious attachment: they phone insistently, exaggerate the gravity of the symptoms, and set up unnecessary appointments. When death occurs, the relatives' expression of hatred reveals itself through resentment, reproach, lawsuits, physical aggression or even murder of the doctor, as has happened in Brazil before.

Terminally ill patients go through the phases of separation in a related manner. Soon after the diagnosis, there is denial[2] of the nearness of death. After getting through this phase, the patient becomes aware of the gravity of the disease and recognizes the possibility of death. Then there is revolt/anger, which, not uncommonly, is directed toward the doctor and/or God. This is followed by sadness, which sometimes leads to depression. Those who are able to get through the previous phases (there are some who remain fixed in them) finally reach acceptance of the inevitable with peace and resignation. Sometimes, at this stage, disturbed relationships are salvaged, making parting with the family more harmonious. The relatives, in turn, also manifest these separation reactions. There is the well-known period of preparing for the loss. For this reason, the mourning period after a sudden loss (in the case of accidents, for example) is, in general, longer and more difficult, and various reactions may occur in an attempt to attenuate the shock. In such cases, the time necessary for the farewell ritual was insufficient.

Concept of self-appreciation

This is considered the *second basic psychodynamic position* in the development of the personality. It begins to function before the birth of the child, as it includes the family's expectations of the new being. This system is responsible for the consciousness of who we are (identity) and how much we are worth (value). It organizes our self-esteem, the perception and elaboration of the esteem that others devote to us. It coordinates, in other words, the dynamics referring to the formation of the self-appreciation concept (family, social, professional, etc.). As with the first basic psychodynamic position, this has two poles. The first refers to the inebriating

---

2 It is common to discover denial of disease in clinical practice. The ill person, as well as his relatives, may deny the symptoms of disease. This denial presents itself with avoidance, delays or procrastination of medical visits. "It is nothing", "It'll cure itself", "It'll go away soon", are phrases that come up. The same thing happens in psychiatry: mystical, religious, or philosophical explanations are developed to cover up the desperation of the official diagnosis. At these times, distant relatives, friends and neighbors manage to see the reality of the situation better than close family can.

sensation that the child experiences when receiving the love of his family group (relationship pole): he/she feels unique and wonderful. This feeling stimulates the desire to show off, as the ego is momentarily inflated.

The second pole represents either the absence or reduction of positive influences or the presence of negative ones – being reprimanded or punished, for example – making the child feel unloved or unadmired by those around him/her (separation): experiencing a lack of love. The child feels low; his/her ego deflates. A *breaking* of the former positive feeling occurs and a *narcissistic wound* (Kohut, 1984) appears. Under these circumstances I add a third possibility: that of the person feeling neither the most beautiful nor the ugliest, but realizing he/she is just average, common. This feeling of not having any special distinction, of not even being a total failure, can bring on the collapse of great yearnings.

The repetition of the bipolar experiences of grandiosity (megalomania) and inferiority (micromania) energetically and emotionally impregnates the personality. An *ideal me* is configured, based on the intoxicating experience of receiving unconditional love and admiration, which leads one to feel that perfection may be reached. The counterpart to the *ideal me* is represented by the *censor me(s)* which criticize in respect to the minimum levels of perfection to be reached. Thus, the *ideal me* serves as a positive parameter in the search for perfection and the perseverance in broadening one's abilities. Yet it also serves as a negative parameter when it becomes a perfectionist compulsion, generating guilt, depression or *narcissistic fury* (Kohut, 1984). This fury may be directed against oneself as well as against those considered guilty of weakness. The counterpart of the *ideal me* is the *un-ideal me*, representing everything the person hopes not to be. As a consequence, in contrast to the ideal (physical–psychological) self-image, there is an un-ideal self-image, whatever the person would hate to be. For a middle-aged person having difficulty accepting getting older, for example, the ideal image would correspond to youth, while the un-ideal image would be senility.[3]

It is important to remember that there are both internal and external self-images.[4] The internal image relates to the functioning of the internal organs. The external refers to the aesthetic self-image. A distorted self-image engenders internal and external hypochondriac aspects. An internal

---

3 Consult "A little incursion into the narcissism of old age" in the book *Gerontodrama: old age on stage* (Costa, 1998).

4 To Brito, self-image "is the totality of internally organized information and evaluations which a person elaborates in respect to his own set of features. It is the vision and form connoted in each person in experiencing his own identity"; or "it is the complex set of information and evaluations which a person forms in respect to himself"; or, still, "the reading that each person does of his own identity from his values, desires and hopes" (1998, pp. 167–169).

hypochondrium corresponds to the classic, obsessive-phobic preoccupation with one's health, the constant fear of getting sick, the attachment to medications, without any treatment being followed to completion.

External (aesthetic) hypochondria is reinforced by the narcissistic times in which we live. The cult of the body, natural diets and exercise clubs reveal the healthy narcissistic facet of our times, but its exaggeration reflects an evident modern hypochondria. By extension, there may be a correct ecology and a hypochondriac one; it is, at times, difficult to distinguish between them. Correct ecology is an appropriate attitude toward preserving the environment. Hypochondriac ecology, however, is seen in fanaticism toward environmental cleanliness expressed by prevalent, persevering, delusional or even delirious ideas.

Babies confuse the *inside* with the *outside* and *partial* with *whole*. He/she responds to partial losses as if they were whole. This happens as much in relation to himself/herself as to others. When the mother removes herself, the baby reacts dramatically, as if he/she were losing his/her mother forever; likewise, when the bathtub is drained, the baby may imagine that he/she will go with the water; when strangers appear suddenly, he/she has a temper tantrum; and so it goes. Some of these reactions remain latent, but may surface in situations of anxiety during adulthood. For example, the hypochondriac extreme represents an exaggeration of a normal reaction. He/she thinks feeling somewhat sick represents total illness which will inevitably lead to death. In attending a person under these circumstances, a doctor must remember that he/she is dealing with both an adult and an (internal) frightened child. Everyone, including the doctor, has a more or less frightened child within him/her. The doctor fears, just like any human being, the molestation of his/her body. In imagining that he/she dominates the other's illness, the doctor may feel in control of his/her own illness as well. In fact, the choice of a medical career clearly indicates a taste for understanding of and dominance over infirmities. In a broad sense, one could say that this *taste for illness* expresses, among other things, a sublimated hypochondriac nucleus.

Triangulation

The third psychodynamic position in the formation of the personality studies the relationships of three people in the *matrix of identity* triangulation. It represents the child's departure from the narrow dual corridor established with his/her caretakers. This is the gateway to future social communication: from the corridor to the triangle, from the triangle to the circle; from the mother to the family, from the family to the social group. Triangulation also shelters the seeds of competition and jealousy.

The *intercessor* may represent someone who saves the child from fusing with the mother, or who steals her from the child. This is a question of timing and intensity of the action. In the intra-uterine life and the first months *post-partum*, the child is protected within the mother's bio-psychological womb. However, remaining in this state means either biological death (delayed delivery) or psychological death (lack of individual identity formation). The *intercessor* promotes the cutting of this symbiotic tie which, while it may have been good before, no longer is. One could even say that, in consecrating this separation, a second birth takes place – a psychological birth, the formation of the identity. A *dis-fusion* of the child's *I* in relation to the mother occurs. The *intercessor* (father) may represent the hero for "executing the cut" at the right time; or, he may symbolize the villain if he fosters the separation before or after the opportune moment. Premature separation corresponds to wrenching apart and delayed separation to suffocation. For a complete analysis, the mother/child, father/child and mother/father dyads, as well as the triangulation among the three within this new relational constellation must be taken into account. The action of the *intercessor* depends, in truth, on the synchronism of the three. Positive resolution of the triangular complex occurs with spontaneous fluency, while the discordant evolution takes place with transferential "bumps".

The figure of the doctor, just like the *intercessor* in the *matrix of identity*, can seem as much a savior as an executioner, depending on the relational synchronism among doctor, patient and health–illness. I don't refer to eventual technical errors, nor to professional unpreparedness, nor to failures in the healthcare system. I focus only on the various psychological shades of the doctor–patient relationship in the psycho(patho)logy of falling ill. For example, one patient receives the technically correct recommendation to operate on a tumor. The doctor states that a hysterectomy is immediately necessary. He doesn't take into consideration that the patient is single and still dreams of having children (nor that the uterus is symbolic of feminine wholeness). The patient, in desperation, looks for another gynecologist – one who reiterates the need for surgery, though accepts that, in order for the patient to get used to the idea, hormones could be prescribed to diminish the bleeding and allow the surgery to be put off. This example reveals the synchronization that the second doctor has with the patient's suffering.

A biblical version of triangulation can be appreciated in Genesis: God (the *intercessor*) *cuts* the tie between the human being (the *first*) and paradise (the *second*), expelling him and her from it.[5] While humans may have gained earthly identity through this act, they also lost their immortal condition and the eternal health they enjoyed in paradise (divine attributes).

---

5 "With sweat, the breathing of your nostrils/you will eat bread/until you render it earth/since from her it was taken/for it is dust and to dust/you will return" (Campos, 1995).

The human being loses unity, receives division. Eternal health becomes health/sickness and eternal life turns to life/death. Oscillation between the two poles becomes man's vital cycle. But man misses the period of *unity*. He/she fantasizes of returning to the previous state of narcissistic plenitude. He/she searches for the magic of returning to paradise through superstitions, quacks and charlatans.

Thus, the doctor not only cares for illness and health, but also works with the health/illness process. Strictly speaking, doctors are not specialized in either health (preventive medicine and public health) or illness (clinical and surgical). The doctor becomes the intercessor in the health/sickness dyad. He confronts the health/sickness process – the *expulsion from paradise syndrome*. In providing a *cure*, he cuts the patient's connection with sickness (death) and saves his/her health (life), as if the patient were returning to paradise where the doctor fulfills the role of God. Because of this temptation the professional must face, he/she may suffer from the *omnipotence–impotence syndrome*, thinking he/she can do either anything or nothing at all.

The third basic psychodynamic position in the formation of the personality, triangulation, deals with the same foundation of the two previous psychodynamic positions: relationship/separation. It rules all of man's movements on earth, including the health/sickness and life/death dyads. In the doctor/patient relationship, the third position is filled by the doctor-patient–health triad or the doctor–patient–illness triad, including their institutional aspects.

The doctor–patient relationship

Doctor and patient establish an unequal or asymmetrical relationship to the extent that the roles that give it structure are different. One possesses technical knowledge; the other doesn't. An asymmetrical relationship differs from an equal or symmetrical one, such as the friend–friend or girlfriend–boyfriend link. There is a qualitative difference, because in the first instance one is there to *receive* care while the other is there to *offer something*. Within an equal relationship, both people give and receive something of the same quality. Obviously, in practice it isn't quite this way. In all relationships, even in asymmetrical ones, there is always giving and receiving, even if in a qualitatively different way. The doctor doesn't receive a cure from the patient, but receives satisfaction from his performance and remuneration for his work. In asymmetrical relationships, one expects to receive something that one doesn't possess or that one wants more of. This peculiarity could suggest that one partner is superior to the other, favoring the appearance of transferential reactions and relationships. Along these lines it is common for a patient to make grandiose projections onto the doctor. Such projections may rouse extreme responses on the part of the professional, either confirming or frustrating them in an inappropriate way.

Study of the doctor–patient relationship during medical school[6] should receive the same level of attention that pharmacology does, since the *medical remedy* is as important as pharmacological drugs. In truth, the ability to "prescribe oneself" in the right dosage at the appropriate time distinguishes a great clinician from a common doctor. Michael Balint (1961) organized groups of English general practitioners and specialists in the hopes that they would be better able to deal with the relationships with their patients.

After having pointed out so many difficulties in the doctor–patient relationship, it may appear that it is always an arduous one. But it isn't. On the contrary, it is most frequently ruled by authentic gratitude, on the one hand, and the genuine happiness of helping, on the other.

References

Abdo, C. H. N. (1996). *Armadilhas da comunicação. O médico, o paciente e o diálogo (Communication traps: the doctor, the patient and the dialogue)*. São Paulo: Lemos.

Balint, M. E. (1961). *El medico, el paciente y la enfermedad*. Buenos Aires: Libros Basicos. (Original edition: *The doctor, his patient and the illness*. London: Sir Isaac Pitman & Sons, 1957.)

Bowlby, J. (1981). *Cuidados maternos e saúde mental*. São Paulo: Martins Fontes. (Original edition: *Child care and the growth of love*. London: Penguin Books Ltd, 1976.)

Brito, D. J. (1998). *Astros e ostras (Stars and oysters)*. São Paulo: Ágora.

Campos, H. (1995). Bereshith: A segunda historia da criação. Astúcia da serpente (The second history of creation. The serpent's guile). *Folha de São Paulo*, May 7: pp. 4–5, 5–6.

Costa, E. S. (1998). *Gerontodrama: a velhice em cena (Gerontodrama: old age on stage)*. São Paulo: Ágora.

Kaufman, A. (1992). *Teatro pedagógico: bastidores da iniciação médica (Pedagogic theater: behind the scenes of medical initiation)*. São Paulo: Ágora.

Kohut, H. (1984). *Self e Narcisismo*. Rio de Janeiro: Zahar Editores S.A. (Original edition: *The search for the self – selected writings of Heinz Kohut – 1950–1978* (2 vols). New York: International Universities Press, Inc., 1978.)

Moreno, J. L. (1974). *Psicoterapia de grupo e psicodrama (Group psychotherapy and psychodrama)*. São Paulo: Mestre Jou. (Original edition: *Gruppenpsychotherapie und psychodrama. Einleitung in die theorie und praxis*. Stuttgart: Georg Thieme Verlag, 1959.)

6 I recommend reading the books: *Pedagogic theater: Behind the scenes of medical initiation* by Arthur Kaufman (1992) and *Communication traps: the doctor, the patient and the dialogue* by Carmita Abdo (1996).

Moreno, J. L. (1977). *Psychodrama – First Volume* (5th edn). New York: Beacon House, Inc.

Winnicott, D. W. (1978). *Da pediatria à psicanálise*. Rio de Janeiro: Francisco Alves. (Original edition: *Collected papers: through paediatrics to psycho-analysis*. London: Tavistock Publications, 1958.)

Chapter 4

Personality diagnosis and identity disorders*

I am what I am

The Lord presenting himself to Moses[1]

The dynamic interaction of the primary and secondary personality characteristics expresses the individual as a whole in his relational world. Even if people cannot be classified from a theoretical-existential point of view (since the human being transcends such classification), from a practical-clinical viewpoint we know that personality disorders are grouped according to certain predominant psychodynamics.

The way in which a child goes through his/her *matrix of identity*[2] forms the parameters of how he/she will turn out as an adult. All of the phases of the matrix are important, although the very first (the *double* and the *mirror* phases, which correspond to the *indifferentiation, symbiosis, recognition of I* and *recognition of you* phases) are definitive in delineating the primary and secondary personality characteristics.

In accordance with the experiences in the *matrix of identity*, groups of people with certain predominant features, characteristics, and psychodynamics can be recognized. Based on Moreno (1977), Kernberg (1979), Kohut (1984) and Fiorini (1985), and from my own observations, I propose four syndrome groups: psychotics, people with identity disorders, neurotics and normotics.[3] Despite the current, especially American (DSM, 1989), psychiatric tendency to pulverize the larger classifications into innumerable small diagnoses, it is worth maintaining these main groups for practical reasons.

---

* Published in the *Brazilian Journal of Psychodrama*, 1995.
1 I am inspired by Muskat (1986, p. 51) who makes this biblical citation in her text on identity.
2 The *matrix of identity* (Moreno, 1977) can be defined as the child's first relational nucleus. This doesn't only mean the two-way mother/child link, but also the emotional result of all the interactions involved in this primary nucleus. Thus the relational network (father–mother, grandparents, aunts and uncles, etc.) surrounding the new being in which biological, physiological and sociocultural factors are intertwined must be taken into consideration.
3 Moreno and Moreno (1964, p. 143).

Normotics, neurotics and psychotics

Normotics represent, for Moreno, people who are neither neurotic nor psychotic. I understand them to be those who constitute the statistical norm, and, therefore, the majority of humanity. I interpret, because Moreno doesn't go into detail, that normotics go through the *matrix of identity* more harmoniously, becoming adults who are more psychologically balanced.

They are distinguished from neurotics, basically, in that they do not present clinical symptoms. By symptom I mean, "the manifestation of an organic or functional alteration perceived by either the doctor or the patient" (Cardenal, 1958). The normotic seeks psychotherapy due to relational, situational or existential difficulties.

In my book *Psychodrama of Madness* (Fonseca, 1980) I introduce the concept of *transferential* (or *psychotic*) *nuclei* of the personality which can be active or dormant. Depending on the degree of difficulty, the personality functions on a *transferential* (or *psychotic*) *level*. *Normotics* present a low level of transference compared to *neurotics*, *psychotics*, and *people with identity disorders* who present, to different degrees and in varied situations, a higher level of transference.

An imbalance of *primary personality traits* combined with the emergence of negative loads foster the appearance of a neurotic profile. In other words, the *neurotic* is an "imbalanced" normotic who, therefore, presents symptoms. Neurotics are commonly characterized by the preponderance of *basic traits* out of balance. In classic terminology, there are obsessives, hysterics and phobics.[4] Detailed clinical observation shows, however, that *neurotics* frequently present a psychoplasticism of combined features: obsessive-phobics or phobic-obsessives and hysterical-phobics or phobic-hystericals. Neurotic shadings of the hypochondriac, depressive or other types are associated in the same way that secondary personality traits are associated to the primary traits described above.

Traditionally, *psychotics* are considered those who present psychotic (delirious and/or hallucinatory) breakdowns. However, one must analyze the individual not only during the psychotic episode, but also outside it, in the "between breakdown" period – the state in which he/she lives the majority of the time. Such observation allows one to verify if and how this psychotic functioning exists. *Normotics*, *neurotics* and *people with identity disorders* may present acute psychotic breakdowns yet easily return to their former state. Other patients do not, functioning with a psychotic personality handicap. In this group, schizophrenias and organic psychoses stand out. *Psychotic dynamics* should also be distinguished from

---

4 For a relational reading on the phobic profile consult Gheller (1992) and Carezzato (1999).

psychotic states. Psychotherapists sometimes confuse a *psychotic dynamic* (which can appear in any patient with the aforementioned symptoms) with a *psychotic state* – a clinical framework structured by specific diagnostic elements.

Identity disorders

Many people who seek psychotherapy don't fit into these descriptions. Observation will reveal that they are people with different characteristics from *normotics*, *neurotics* and *psychotics*. I refer to this group (known in the literature as people with narcissistic disorders, immature personalities, character neuroses, people with personality disorders, psychopaths and pathological narcissism) as *people with identity disorders.*[5] According to Fiorini (1985), the wolf man and the rat man, presented as neurotics by Freud (Notes Upon a Case of Obsessional Neurosis), could be included in this new category. These manifestations originate in the phase of identity construction; that is, the *recognition of I phase* or the *mirror phase* in the matrix of identity. *Identity* formation is understood as the process by which the child "un-fuses" himself from the *undifferentiated chaos* from which he/ she came, gaining consciousness of himself (*singularity*) and of the other (*alterity*), through the connections (in their two polarities: relation/ separation) established in his/her matrix of identity. This process begins in the *matrix of identity*, beginning with the identity of *I*, and continues throughout life with the search for the *profound I* or the *real I*.

People with identity disorders traverse the *matrix of identity* in an impaired way. Characteristically, they adopt a number of shock absorbers (defenses) that, as a whole, are insufficient for the harmonious functioning of the personality.

In a certain phase of the *matrix of identity*, the baby experiences the sensation that he/she is beautiful, loved and admired. As Kohut (1984) says, the child registers "the shine in his mother's eyes". This energetic impregnation develops and imprints a sensation of grandiosity and exhibitionism in the child. On the other hand, when this experience fails to happen, the child senses the loss of these inebriating feelings, becoming immersed in the pain provoked by this *narcissistic wound* (Kohut, 1984). The balance or imbalance of this duality (relationship/separation, love/rejection, pleasure/ pain) separates healthy self-esteem and tolerance toward frustration from

---

5 For a broader study, I suggest the book *Emotional survival* by Rosa Cukier (1998). I also recommend the articles "Narcissistic and borderline disorders: a permeable border?" by Teodoro Herranz Castillo (1996), "Feelings of hate in marcissism" by Vera Rolim (1997) and "Narcissism – the first universe" by Carlos Calvente (1999).

pathological identity disorders. In this phase, the child gains the sometimes painful understanding that he/she is not always special – the best or the worst – but only average or mediocre.[6]

The rudiments of the *ideal I* – always be loved and admired – appear in contrast to the *I* that doesn't receive these positive inputs. In terms of development, this is the beginning of the *be/appear* dyad: "If I am not what I would like to be, then I will try to appear to be." The *self-image* is either fixed or obscured, depending on the inputs received from the *other*. It becomes distinguished from or confused with the *ideal you* (who praises) or the *frustrating you* (who criticizes).[7]

The upheaval involved during the formation of the *self-worth concept* of the personality is seen in insecure people who present accented relational difficulties and the consequent suffering of both themselves and those with whom they are involved. They present serious difficulties fitting in, both socially and professionally. In the psychological and psychopathological expression of identity disorders, a large variety of features, signs and symptoms appear: anxiety, eccentricity, dramaticism, hysteria, schizoid features, anti-social attitudes, paranoid, phobic, obsessive-compulsive and depressive elements and passive–aggressive and dependent manifestations. These patients frequently succumb to drug use, seeking a chemical crutch for their hobbled personalities.

The prevailing questions for these people are: who am I?; what am I worth?; how do I appear to others? In this sense, the illness is the self-doubt itself. The poorly delineated self-image oscillates between grandiosity and catastrophic devaluation. *People with identity disorders* alternate between the *ideal I* and the *I* (considered a failure) – they are either the best or the worst. They search for confirmation of their existence and self-worth through the eyes of the other. They aren't genuinely interested in the *other*, but in his applause. They depend on people who are significant to them and complement them narcissistically. Wounded in the matrix of identity, they try to reduce their pain through compensatory relational dynamics but frequently succumb to the disorganized ups and downs of guilt, depression, shame and fury (Kohut, 1984). Depression and guilt originate from their unfulfilled grandiose ideas.

Clinically, three types of guilt can be distinguished: schizoid, reparative and narcissistic or "*I*-ist". In schizoid guilt, the individual believes that the bad is within him/her, that he/she is intrinsically bad. Harming *the other* is

6 *Mediocris* from Latin: "that which is neither good nor bad, or that is between good and bad; that which is neither large nor small" (Candido de Figueiredo, 1947).

7 In the construction of identity, various categories are involved which I distinguish as *I*, *self-image*, *ideal I*, *partial Is*, *censoring Is* and *profound I* or *real I*. In considering the structuring of the identity as an imminently relational process, I also give weight to the concepts of *you* or *other*, *ideal you* and *frustrating you*.

an automatic occurrence in the relationship; through *the other*, the schizoid is conscious of his/her "badness". This leads him/her to avoid relational situations, isolating him/herself, in order to be spared these painful feelings. Reparative guilt stems from the recognition of one's hate toward a *frustrating you* and to the moral/ethical conscience that he/she has hurt another. This consciousness leads him/her to ask for forgiveness. Narcissistic guilt refers to the hatred turned against oneself for not having reached *ideal* performance. The intensity of the guilt suggests its healthy or pathological connotation. Along these lines, *innate* or *existential guilt*, about which Buber (1957) speaks, mustn't be forgotten. For Buber, guilt, regardless of neurosis or psychosis, is an inherent human feeling, making the acceptance of errors an element inseparable from the truth.

Depression and narcissistic guilt have a dual relational structure – that is, the confrontation of the *ideal I* with the *I*. Shame, which also has a narcissistic connotation, contains a triadic structure in that it includes the look of the *other* in the real/ideal comparison. Shame is self-deception in the presence of the *other*. A weakness which was formerly internal (psychological), and therefore private, is exposed (social) and moves to the public dominion.

Depressive characteristics of identity disorders contain aggression toward others uncommon in other depressive states. *Ideal you(s)* disappoint simply by being *you(s)*, becoming *frustrating you(s)*, susceptible to aggression. *Fury* is an inward or outward aggressive expression when the idealized self-image collapses. *People with identity disorders*, fearing the rupture of their self-image, present paranoid sensitivity and self-regarding features: what do they think of me?; don't they like me?

The *global I* is made up of innumerable *partial I(s)*. The inability to apprehend this structure leads to confusing the *partial I* with the *global I*. An observation referring to the *partial* may be understood as referring to the *global*, often manifested by an extreme sensitivity to criticisms.

Doubt about self-image invades all the relational fields. Insecurity is also reflected in the apprehension of the *bodily I*. The *bodily I* refers to the physiological consciousness of the internal organs (physiological self-image). The *external bodily I* rules the consciousness of the external body (aesthetic self-image); that is, the way the individual perceives himself externally. As "health" is classically defined as the *silence of the organs*, it can be said that people with identity disorders present "noises", which are manifested by psychosomatic disorders and obsessive aesthetic and hypochondriac ruminations. As Winnicott (1990) says, the problem for hypochondriacs is their doubt about illness, not the illness itself. In the same way, dysfunctions, doubts and unsatisfactions occur in the sexual sphere. Sexual identity disorders appear in two spheres: the gender sexual identity (am I a man or a woman?) and the relational sexual identity, the definition of sexual attraction (who am I attracted to?). People with sexual identity disorders present a vast array of manifestations which include gender identity disorders, sadomasochist pathologies and sexual dysfunction.[8]

The unstable organization of psychological shock absorbers (defenses) in *people with identity disorders* leads to hysterical, phobic and obsessive *primary traits*, uncommon in *neurotics* and *normotics*. In these, the predominant combination is of two (of the three cited) primary neurotic traits. In *people with identity disorders*, other traits may emerge, depending on the level of anxiety, forming a kaleidoscope of signs and symptoms.

Classification[9]

Depending on the predominant traits, signs and symptoms (though they frequently appear mixed), identity disorders are grouped into psychosomatic illnesses, sexual identity disorders, people with false I or "as if" personalities, psychopathies and borderline personalities (with psychotics).

Psychosomatic illnesses include the profound disorders of the *bodily I* (internal and external) manifested through a variety of clinical profiles such as anorexia and bulimia; certain types of rheumatism; the poli-operated syndrome (also mistakenly referred to as the Munchausen syndrome) in which patients induce their (uniformed) doctors to operate on them innumerable times; some chronic gastrointestinal disorders, etc. One must hesitate, however, before accepting an illness as psychosomatic, as there exists a tendency in medicine to label all clinical profiles of unclarified etiology as such.

Sexual identity disorders represent distortions of the *sexual I* – doubts and anxieties over the (in)definition of the sexual identity. These cover the clinical profiles otherwise referred to in the psychoanalytic literature as sexual perversions.

People with *false I* or *"as if" personalities* represent the *ideal I* figure in the internal theater of their minds. But this *false I* is fragile and succumbs to the introduction of life's natural resistances. The *false I* functions like a shell over the *real I*; when the shell breaks, depression or psychosis emerges.

Psychopaths[10] are also called *actuators*. This category includes people who are characterized by an insufficient capacity to assume guilt and whose muscular *armour* is inadequate to control internal, especially aggressive, impulses. Since the intensity of this trait varies, people ranging from the abnormal (in a statistical sense) but not pathological, to the frankly

---

8 See Part 3, "Psychodrama and Sexuality".

9 I follow the classification used by Fiorini (1985) with few alterations: I include the psychopath subgroup and denominate as *sexual identity disorders* what he calls *sexual perversions*.

10 I conserve the denomination *psychopath* for the fact that despite the prejudices contained within it and by those intent on substituting it, it is a consecrated term.

pathological, can be included. Thus, many criminals are classified here, but some men of social success could also be included.

Borderline personalities are difficult to differentiate from psychotics. Observing the evolution of "outbreak" and "between-break" periods over the years permits appropriate diagnosis. In addition to basic doubts concerning their relational and existential identity, *borderline personalities* demonstrate great emotional instability, oscillating between delirious states and psychotic anxiety and depression. Psychotic breaks come and go with the same ease.

All people construct an identity and, therefore, experience the existential vicissitudes described here. The psychodynamics of *identity disorders*, in truth, pertain to all human beings. What distinguishes *people with identity disorders*, who markedly aggregate these described characteristics, is the complex fact of having suffered more, by internal/external conditions, in the identity formation period and their desperate search in the present for what they were unable to get in the past. I want to emphasize that a pathological condition follows a gradual scale of intensity. At one extreme, we find the normal characteristics of the trait, at the other the pathological. With *identity disorders*, the manifestations are massive and more painfully evident.

References

Buber, M. (1957). Guilt and guilt feelings. The William Alanson White Lectures. Fourth series. *Psychiatry*, 20, 2.

Calvente, C. (1999) Narcisismo – primer universo (Narcissism – the first universe). Oral communication. II Ibero-American Congress of Psychodrama, Águas de São Pedro, SP.

Cardenal, L. (1958). *Dicionário terminológico de ciências médicas (Dictionary of medical sciences terminology)*. Barcelona: Salvat.

Carezzato, M. C. (1999). Uma leitura psicodramática da síndrome de pânico (A psychodramatic reading of panic syndrome). *Revista Brasileira de Psicodrama*, 7, 2.

Cukier, R. (1992). *Psicodrama bipessoal (Bi-personal psychodrama)*. São Paulo: Ágora.

Cukier, R. (1998). *Sobrevivência emocional (Emotional survival)*. São Paulo: Ágora.

Figueiredo, C. (1947). *Dicionário da língua portuguesa (Portuguese language dictionary)*. Lisboa: Bertrand-Jackson.

Fiorini, H. J. (1985). Notes from the course "Narcissistic disorders". Daimon-Centro de Estudos do Relacionamento, São Paulo.

Fonseca, J. (1980). *Psicodrama da loucura (Psychodrama of madness)*. São Paulo: Ágora.

Gheller, J. H. (1992). Síndrome do pânico: visão psicodinâmica–relacional–psicodramática (Panic syndrome: a psychodynamic–relational–psychodramatic view). *Psicodrama, Revista da SOPSP*, 4.

Herranz Castillo, T. (1996) Transtornos narcisista y borderline: ¿Una frontera permeable? (Narcissistic and borderline disorders: A permeable border?). *Revista Brasileira de Psicodrama*, 4, fascículo II.

Kernberg, O. F. (1979). *Desórdenes fronterizos y narcisismo patológico*. Buenos Aires: Paidós. (Original edition: *Borderline conditions and pathological narcissism*. New York: Jason Aronson, 1975.)

Kohut, H. (1984). *Self e narcisismo*. Rio de Janeiro: Zahar. (Original edition: *The search for the self – Selected writings of Heinz Kohut: 1950–1978* (2 vols). New York: International Universities Press, Inc., 1978.)

McCord, W. and McCord, J. (1966). *El psicópata. (The psychopath)*. Buenos Aires: Hormé.

Manual de diagnóstico e estatística de distúrbios mentais (DSM-III-R) (1989). São Paulo: Manole, 3rd ed. (Original edition: *Diagnostic and statistical manual of mental disorders. DSM-III-R*. Washington, DC: American Psychiatric Press, 1987.)

Mayer-Gross, W., Slater, E. and Roth, M. (1972). *Psiquiatria clínica*. São Paulo: Mestre Jou. (Original edition: *Clinical psychiatry*. London: Baillière, Tindall & Cassell Ltd, 1954, 1960, 1969.)

Moreno, J. L. (1977). *Psychodrama – First Volume* (5th edn). New York, Beacon House.

Moreno, J. L. and Moreno, Z. J. (1964). *The first psychodramatic family*. New York: Beacon House, Inc.

Muskat, M. (1986). *Consciência e identidade (Consciousness and identity)*. São Paulo: Ática.

Rolim, V. (1997). Sentimento de ódio no narcisismo (Feelings of hate in narcissism). *Revista Brasileira de Psicodrama*, 5, 2.

Schneider, K. (1965). *Las personalidades psicopáticas (The psychopathic personalities)*. Madrid: Morata.

Winnicott, D. W. (1990). *Natureza humana*. Rio de Janeiro: Imago. (Original edition: *Human nature*. London: Free Association, 1988.)

Part 2

New approaches to psychodrama technique

Chapter 5

Individual psychotherapy and psychodrama

Relationship psychotherapy

In this chapter I will be describing the approach to individual psycho-therapy that I have been using for some years. This method emerged spontaneously, nourished by theoretical and methodological influences that occurred throughout my career. At a certain point I noticed that my perspective was neither that of psychoanalytical psychotherapy nor of psychodrama. Nevertheless, psychodrama has clearly influenced my methodology.

The term *relationship psychotherapy* refers to a type of psychotherapy that deals with both the client–therapist relationship and the relationships from the client's internal world (*I–you* and *I–I* relationships). Relationship psychotherapy is also the term that some German psychotherapists, such as von Weizsäcker and Trub gave to psychotherapy based on the philosophy of Martin Buber.

Regardless of the orientation, client and therapist participate in a human encounter and take on different roles. The client is searching for help; the therapist is at the client's service. This creates a connection that defines the basis of their relationship founded on non-egalitarian roles. Despite this inequality, the participants form a horizontal relationship within a common psychological space – the *inter*. The therapeutic *inter* is necessary for the development of the process of *being*, in contrast to *appearing*. Knowing how to create these circumstances is, for the therapist, a more innate than learned process.

When an individual's personality begins to develop (in the *matrix of identity*) it is structured into several *main* traits, along with a number of secondary ones. The *arrangement* (or structure) of these traits defines the basic characteristics of the individual. The traits possess both a positive and a negative side, where *shock absorbers* (defenses) are located. For example, an obsessive client presents – on the positive side – elements of reflection, organization, planning, cleaning, etc., and – on the negative side – over-intellectualization, mental rumination, affective distancing, compulsion for order and cleanliness, obsessive doubting, etc. The overall goal is to search for harmony of functioning. The *main traits* do not change; they are the individual's trademarks. The therapist attempts, however, to work through the negative burdens and liberate the positive potential inherent to the trait. While the therapeutic approach toward the *main traits* is an important point in psychotherapy, it is not the only point.

Relationship psychotherapy starts with pragmatic observation and comprehension of the relationship phenomenon. The diagnosis (in the sense of knowledge) of *inter* is the way to attain the diagnosis of oneself, or consciousness of oneself (*I*). The development of the *I observer*, which leads the distorted self-image to become a true *I*, is a primary goal. The *I observer* is a third eye which does not judge, criticize or praise; instead, it witnesses. The *I* is formed by a complex of internalized *partial I(s)* that shout out to be discovered and that express themselves through role-playing.

Relationship psychotherapy always alternates among three perspectives. It is either centered on the client (that is, on his life relationships), on the client–therapist relationship, or on the therapist, in the sense that the therapist receives, feels and responds therapeutically. I believe that the first two perspectives require no explanation. To illustrate a situation in which the session can focus on the personal attitudes of the therapist, I offer the following example. A patient who misses sessions or constantly arrives late might receive the following assessment: "Regardless of my ability to comprehend the reasons for your absences, I must say that it is difficult for me to relate to a person like this. It is a little frustrating. Is it possible that the people in your relationships also feel this way? If they do not, it is because they complement your fear of diving in, of submitting yourself to a relationship."

The relationship psychotherapist is a blend of psychodrama director and auxiliary ego – a therapeutic actor, so to speak. Thus, knowledge of both psychodynamics and psychodramatic training is required. Of course, the better the therapist is able to flow with the technique, the more advantageous the "dramatic quality" will be (by dramatic quality I refer to one of the components of spontaneity, according to Moreno). The scenes are played verbally, with the therapist enacting the internalized roles of the patient. The situations are played primarily in the *here and now*. There is no stage. There is no physical interaction between therapist and client (i.e., no touching during the action). The therapist tries to avoid transferential induction, or an unnecessary emotional commitment. In classical psychodrama the action occurs between the protagonist and the auxiliary ego, with the director at a distance. This necessary distance is preserved in relationship psychotherapy by the therapist playing roles but not physically involving him/herself in the scenes. If and when any physical contact does occur it should not be distorted by other roles that are not inherent to the basic therapist–client situation. In other words, to avoid confusing the client, the therapist should only touch the client in the role of him/herself as therapist, and not as an internalized role of the patient.

The therapist's playing of the client's internalized roles, rather than being confusing, actually permits an easier discrimination among these figures and the real figure of the therapist (at least for patients not experiencing a psychotic episode). Any transferences that do occur become better *visualized* by the therapist.

Relationship psychotherapy does not attempt to instigate transference. This does not mean that I am against the appearance of transference. On the contrary, it is a rich opportunity, a live journey that permits the client to expand the understanding and consciousness of his/her interior world. My expectation, however, is that transference ought to arise naturally, in an unpremeditated fashion. We know that the psychotherapeutic process, through its length and repeated contact, leads to transitory transference reactions or transferential neurosis. Both possibilities are worked through by returning to the *telic* space. *Telic* space can be defined as the virtual space that contains a reciprocal relationship. Investigation of transference is one aspect of therapeutic work. Work within the *telic* space is another moment. Conditions exist within the *telic* space to work with internalized transferential relationships or "auto-transference". However, the point is to achieve "auto-tele" (the greatest *telic* level possible in relation to internal figures). A *working alliance* (Greenson, 1982) inserts itself in the *telic* space.

The therapist conducts him/herself according to the *double principle* (that is, to be in *telic* harmony and realize and/or express what the client needs but is unable to obtain alone) and by the *surrender principle* that leads us to consider news ways of resolving the same problem in respect to the role played. The relationship therapist should put aside theoretical hypotheses, and simply dive into the role being played. This way, everything captured from the client will flow both consciously and unconsciously. Beyond the conscious–conscious contact there is also unconscious–unconscious contact (co-conscious and co-unconscious from Moreno). In this manner, the therapist believes in his *internal operational model* (Greenson, 1982). I believe that in psychodramatic role-play there is a process similar to the incorporation of Candomblé and Umbanda,[1] except that these have religious explanations. I believe that in both situations an altered state of consciousness occurs which facilitates *co-unconscious communication*.

Many times after a role-play, I am surprised with things I had already known, but hadn't realized I knew, about the client. Furthermore, simply role-playing, in and of itself (without concern about the content), is invigorating for the participants. I believe that, while playing the role of

---

1 Candomblé and Umbanda are African-Brazilian religious sects that induce altered states of consciousness through songs, dances and repeated percussion sounds as one of their rituals. In these states, some participants (mediums) "receive" the spirits of African entities (gods/goddesses).

another person and even only partially letting go of my own identity to receive the other's identity, and then returning to myself, subtle alterations in states of consciousness occur, liberating energy that is manifested by a sense of well-being, or even a light euphoria.

The objective is to transform *repetition compulsion*[2] into *differentiated repetition.*[3] For this to happen, the therapeutic procedures are also repeated. One of the client's particular relationships may be the object of various scenes played. Enlarging one's consciousness of the conflict helps to leave the conflict *in spiral,* with each experience increasing the spin upwards.

As in Gestalt therapy, the questions *what?, how?* and *what for?* are prioritized; I add the question *why not?* because this leads us to consider new ways of resolving the same problem. The question *why?* incites explanations and excuses, and invites us to return to our past and to intellectualizations. The answer *because* may be the natural occurrence of a therapeutic action, but never a goal in itself. The presentation of evidence precedes the explanation. This does not mean that the therapist can never ask *why?* or answer *because,* but this represents an attitude in which the present is emphasized.

A psychotherapeutic process consists of the initial interviews and the sessions that follow. These sessions are the psychotherapy itself. The interviews consist of initial contacts that focus on beginning the therapeutic work. The interviews, from a didactic point of view, are divided into four phases: *study* or *diagnosis, planning, commitment* and *contract.* Depending on the professional, there could be various interviews or only one. These phases intertwine. Each of the four phases occurs reciprocally, in that the therapist applies them to the client and vice versa. The *study* or *diagnosis phase* is initiated when the client sets up the first interview; it continues with the first handshake, and proceeds with verbalizing the motive for consultation and the primary complaints. Diagnosing must be understood here not as labeling but as getting to know each other through the relationship. The therapist comes to realize the type of person that he/she has before him/her and what the client's psychodynamic characteristics are. The client studies and "diagnoses" the therapist to see if he/she inspires trust.

The *planning phase* develops while study or diagnosis is still taking place. The therapist begins to formulate a work plan. The client also has a plan – to get better. By comparing both goals, a definitive plan is formed. In the third phase, the *commitment phase,* the degree of commitment from both client and therapist to the long and arduous work ahead is determined. It is better not to initiate the process when doubts remain regarding commitment; it is

2 "Repetition compulsion", expression coined by Freud.
3 "Differentiated repetition", expression used by Fiorini (1978).

therapeutic to instigate a clearer commitment when one does not appear. Having surpassed the three previous phases, a traditional *work contract* is made in order to meet both the therapist's and client's needs.

The final part of the psychotherapeutic process may occur in three ways: *abandonment*, *stop* and *conclusion*. I make this distinction to suggest three different psychodynamic contents and, hence, three approaches as well. *Abandonment* consists of interruption of the process due to transferential elements. In general, it is a brusque rupture, without the opportunity to elaborate on the breaking of the bond. There is a high level of anxiety, which brings discomfort to the client, therapist and group (in the case of group psychotherapy). We cannot forget that separation is a human being's greatest psychological pain. Separation is one of the poles of the relationship/separation pair where at one extreme we have relationship/life and at the other separation/loss/death. Thus, these situations are an invitation for the people involved (including the therapist) to act in transferential roles. The *stop* represents an interruption of the process due to physical or geographical reasons (moves, scheduling conflicts, etc.). In such cases, a long-distance *telic* link remains, which creates the possibility for psychotherapy to resume when circumstances permit again.

The *conclusion* is the closure of a circular movement that has a beginning, middle and end. The psychodynamic elaboration of separation occurs. The environment is *telic*. There is agreement that it is time to leave. Sadness, which is more a sensation of missing the other, always exists, but happiness and satisfaction prevail.

The action *processes* for relationship psychotherapy (Bustos, 1979) contain two parts. The verbal part is made up of the common psychoanalytical psychotherapy actions that attempt to provide, or amplify, insights for the reconstruction of the self-image, or the *telic* perception of the surrounding world. This happens within the verbal context of the session itself or after a *dramatic* action.[4]

In the context of the *dramatic* action, dramatic insight and catharsis of integration present themselves as therapeutic action *processes*. Insight occurs during the playing of a scene and reflects the illumination of a certain problem. Catharsis of integration consists of disorganizing the conflict structure that results in a reorganization, more *telic* than the first.

Whenever possible, both the verbal part and the dramatic action occur in a "playful" space; this is the intermediary zone between the outside and the

---

4 In relationship psychotherapy, I prefer to use the expression *dramatic action* to distinguish it from *dramatization* (*drama–action*) of classical psychodrama. The *dramatic* action does not use the *mise-en-scène*, or corporeal movement of classical psychodrama. The *dramatic action* is a psychodramatic incursion in the verbal context of the session. As in *dramatization*, *dramatic action* presents three movements: introduction, development and resolution.

inside, between the consciousness and the unconsciousness of the client and therapist; in other words, of the therapeutic relationship. This "playful" environment, which the therapist should know how to create, is where insight takes place (see transitional phenomenon, space, and object, from Winnicott, 1975).

Last but not least, there remains *internalization of the therapeutic relationship model* as a *mechanism* of therapeutic action. The internalization of this relationship happens within the molds of other internalized matrices of life (family, school, seminary, religious groups, military services, etc.). The primary *matrix of identity* is the most potent, but the secondary matrices leave marks on the personality also. Some issues can be *re-matricized*,[5] and this characteristic gives strength to the psychotherapeutic process.

The technical aspects of relationship therapy must also be attended to. The setting is the same as with verbal psychotherapies: in a room, with two chairs, one in front of the other. In the verbal context of the session, one operates with the traditional instruments of psychoanalytical psychotherapy: colloquial interaction, *signs* and interpretations (Bustos, 1979). *Signs* may range from indications about the verbal material to body *signs* (physical posture, gestures, tone of voice, look, etc.), referring to the client's form of expression. Since, as the saying goes, "the unconscious is on the face", many unconscious signs are revealed through bodily manifestations. These *signs* lead to self-interpretation by the client, without taking the therapist into account. *Interpretation*, as it is classically conceived, refers to the therapist's acting to make conscious what is unconscious, or make more conscious what is partially conscious.

The theme of the session could be in the *then and there* or in the *here and now*. In the former, the analysis focuses on the relationships of the client in his "outside" life, and in the latter on the relationship with the therapist, here "inside". From the existential point of view, the *here and now* always underlies a recounting of the *then and there*. The therapist has one eye on the *there* and the other on the *here*. Relationship psychotherapy preserves the value of pair sociometry, devalued by Moreno in favor of group sociometry. But group sociometry is used in the study of the *internal group* of the client.

There are diverse technical procedures relative to the *dramatic* action. While the majority of the techniques presented here are derived from psychodrama, some are from Gestalt therapy. As already indicated, classical psychodrama techniques have been simplified. They have been adapted to the 50 minutes of an individual psychotherapy session in contrast to the

---

5 Expression used by the author in his book *The psychodrama of madness* (Fonseca, 1980).

120 minutes of a group psychotherapy session. They have become quicker and more agile. Stage markings are not used to set up the scene; the characters to be role-played frequently "come" to the setting; chronological time is not delineated; nor does spatial movement exist in the *role reversal*. A succession of dramatic actions can occur, leaving time for verbal elaborations. Relationship psychotherapy uses "guerrilla warfare" tactics: actions that are quick and focused on the main goal; surprise attacks and retreats; return to the base for evaluation; and new skirmishes with light weapons, easy to recharge. Classical psychodrama, in comparison, uses "classical war" techniques: heavy weaponry, potent but cumbersome to move. Classical psychodrama works better in the "battlefield" of group psychotherapy. Relationship psychotherapy is more appropriate for the "jungle" of individual psychotherapy.

In the description of techniques that follows, I have left out detailed explanations since they are already familiar to psychodramatists.

The use of the *double technique* and the *mirror technique* are synthesized in relationship psychotherapy in the *double-mirror*. When I employ this technique, which I do frequently, I face the client, doubling him/her. In this way, it is characterized as both a *mirror* and a *double-mirror*.

Role-playing is the procedure most frequently used. I either assume one of the client's internalized roles, previously performed by him, or I perform the role directly, molding myself in accordance with the interaction. This, of course, requires practice. For example, I could say, "I'm your father. Talk to me." In the second role play I could say: "You are your father and I am you." Loosely speaking, we are using *role reversal*. (Strictly speaking, *role reversal* only happens when the therapist and client reverse their own roles as themselves.) Sometimes I use the *interview technique*; in other words, I interview the character incorporated by the client.

The *concretion technique* of sensations and feelings is also frequently used. This happens through body postures or through the placement and pressure of the client's hands over regions of his own body. The *maximization technique* consists of accentuating or exacerbating the concretions. The *repetition technique* consists, as the name itself states, of the repetition of determined verbal expressions or of the repetition of the individual's spontaneous movements. It can be performed in slow motion or fast motion. It is worth emphasizing the unconscious content underlying these expressions. The therapist can also make the person more sensitive, in order to visualize new scenes with a more evident psychodynamic content.

The *presentification technique* corresponds to *dramatization* in classic psychodrama (Perls began to use this technique inspired from theatre and psychodrama). The client is asked to relate the scene in the present, as opposed to the past. The emotion is "presentified" and the therapist includes him/herself in the situation, engaging in dialogue with the client. For example, a dream would normally be related in the past:

"I was in a cave."
"And I was scared."

With *presentification* we would have:

"I'm in a cave."
"What's it like?"
"It's dark and hot."
"How are you feeling?"
"Fine, and bad. I'm afraid, but at the same time there is something pleasant."
"Let's see which part of your body has fear and which part of your body has pleasure."

And so it continues in this manner. *Presentification* can be *centered* or *in the mirror*. In the first case, the person is in the scene, in action, and narrating from this standpoint. In the second case, the individual sees him/herself in the scene and relates from outside. *Centered presentification* is told in the first person (I). *Presentification in the mirror* could be in the first person (I) or the third person singular (he, she). These two possibilities can enrich the psychodramatic work of the scene. The *centered* form corresponds to the relationship and the *mirrored* form to distance. *Relationship* and *distance* permit two different perspectives of the interpersonal relationship. Sometimes I use *soliloquy* during *presentification*.

"You are the cave. What are you like?"
"I'm dark, hard, hot, etc."

Presentification realized with the eyes closed and through the visualization of the scene is called the *videotape technique*. This can also be *centered* or *mirrored*. *Videotape* is a technique founded in *internal psychodrama* (visualization of internal images). I distinguish between *videotape* and *internal psychodrama* in that the former refers to an immediate visualization of meaningful scenes from the patient's life. I say: "Close your eyes and visualize the situation." I prefer to use the term *internal psychodrama* for a procedure realized when the person does not have specific material to work with. It is like a trip, an adventure through the unconscious via spontaneous visual images. This trip requires previous preparation for relaxation and concentration. It develops in a more defined state of consciousness than that of the *videotape technique*.

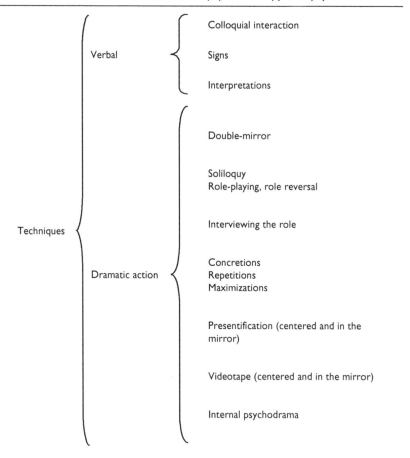

Role-play, role reversal, double-mirror and videotape

The following dialogue, taken from a session with one of my patients, demonstrates these techniques:

T: You visualized a scene in which you are with a man you're interested in but act as if you aren't. And you said that you've frequently shown this attitude in your life. I propose that I be this man for a few minutes. What is his name?

P: Roberto.

T: I'll be Roberto; you'll be able to speak with him here. When I'm going to stop being Roberto, I'll let you know, OK?

P: OK.

Role-play technique

T:	[Roberto]: I've shown up in your scene and I'm here to talk. What would you like to tell me?
P:	Roberto . . . I feel like . . . getting closer to you . . . and getting closer . . . without pretending.
Roberto:	You're pretending?
P:	Sometimes I pretend to be indifferent . . . I disguise what I'm feeling.
Roberto:	I wonder if it's possible for a man and a woman to get close without any games.
P:	Good question.
Roberto:	Do you think that you're playing games, that I am, or that we both are?
P:	We both are.
Roberto:	How do you see me in the situation? What do you think about the way I am?
P:	You're afraid of me.
Roberto:	How do you know? What makes you feel this? What about your fear? What are you afraid of?
P:	Rejection. Roberto, I can't stand seeing that face you're making!
Roberto:	When you stare at me that way I feel a little uncomfortable. You stare like this . . .
P:	This is what you're afraid of! But this is the way I am.
Roberto:	You are the way you are and I am the way I am.
P:	What am I going to do?
Roberto:	What are we going to do?
P:	The only choice left . . . is to pretend that I'm not like that . . . and be like this . . .
T:	[returning to his role]: Let's reverse roles. You don't need to move. You switch to being Roberto and I'll be you.

Technique of role reversal

T/[Patient]:	This is what I was saying, Roberto . . . I pretend. I pretend when I'm with you because . . .
P/[Roberto]:	You pretend?
T/P:	I pretend, I make a face like this, look away, disguise . . .
P/R:	I never thought you were a fake.
T/P:	I'm not a fake like that. I hide my desire . . . my interest in you . . . do you understand?
P/R:	I don't want pretence.

T/P:	But if I don't pretend, you get scared. Just my staring at you makes you afraid. I'm afraid of being rejected . . . I'm afraid that you don't want me. This is why I pretend. But since I'm not pretending today, can I ask you a direct question? What, really, do you feel for me? You can tell me; I can take it.
P/R:	I admire you, but I don't love you. I prefer a gentler woman, a sweeter woman, for someone to love.
T:	[returning to his role]: Let's go back to the previous roles. You go back to being you and I'll be Roberto again.

Role-play technique

(R):	So, I really admire you; I think you're a great person. But I prefer a gentler, a sweeter women. I prefer a woman who's more receptive to me. Now, I don't know if my saying this hurts . . .
(P):	[Remains in silence, turns her head away and looks down and stays this way]
T:	[returning to his role]: Let's cut this role-play. I'll go back to being the therapist and you continue as the patient. How are you feeling? What feeling do you have in your body?
P:	[Remains in silence]
T:	Let's do patient and patient talking to each other now, as if you were in front of a mirror.

Double-mirror technique

T/P:	So, how are you feeling? We're direct and see what happens? It seems as if men don't like straightforward women. He was afraid of us. He wants someone sweet, someone foolish. And here we are once again, looking at each other. What do you say to me? We've been together for so long . . .
P:	I don't know what to do.
T/P:	Me neither.
P:	We've been together for a long time, and it was such a long road that led us to being direct . . . The price was high . . . but I like it.
T/P:	We've paid a high price for being direct and we like being this way, but it really hurts.
P:	And sometimes I'm not . . . But every time I'm not direct, I regret it later . . .
T/P:	If we're too direct, we push people away.
P:	And if we aren't direct . . . we pretend and nothing happens. And we wind up alone.

T/P:	What happens? I wonder if the men are wrong, or is it that we do something wrong? Do you think it would be possible to change something?
P:	I'm open to change.
T/P:	But change what? Let's pretend that we've changed?
P:	A change to pretending – this I don't want. I'm tired of being alone. You too.
T/P:	Really tired. Now I ask myself: how is it that we learned to be this way?
P:	It was with Dad.
T:	Very good. We'll cut here and let's talk with Dad. I'm the father and you're you – right here and now, at your present age.

Role-play technique

T/[Father]:	My daughter, you've asked me here . . . What do you want?
P:	Oh, Dad . . . you left me an "inheritance" . . . You taught me so much, to do things right . . .
F:	Sure.
P:	To be honest.
F:	Of course.
P:	To not tell lies.
F:	Right . . . and?
P:	Dad, do you love me?
F:	Why are you asking me this? I taught you all these things, left this "inheritance" . . . What is your doubt?
P:	I hope that you love me. I did everything you wanted!
F:	Did you do everything to please me?
P:	Yes, I did!
F:	If you did everything to please me, why do you doubt that I love you?
P:	When I was little, you didn't love me. You only started loving me when I became strong . . .
F:	You started to do everything to please me, to be the way I said you had to be.
P:	When I was a weak little girl, you liked my sister more. I don't know if I won your love or your admiration. Admiration I know I won.
T:	Let's reverse roles. You'll be the father and I'll be you.

Technique of role reversal

T/P: Look, Dad, I did exactly everything you wanted and I became the person you wanted me to be. You liked direct and strong people . . . And I became all this to please you. Because, deep down, I was weak; I had insecurities, fear – but you didn't like me this way. I sensed that you didn't love me.

P/F: My daughter, I taught you all this because life is hard. Otherwise, life would have defeated you.

T/P: What did I get out of this? Did I get you to love me? I ask you now – did you love me, Dad?

P/F: I'm proud of you.

T/P: I always suspected this . . . that, deep down, you only admired me . . . but I'm not sure I ever received the love I've looked for my whole life. I had to change my very essence. I used to be different. It's just that I was a child and I thought: I have to be the way he wants. And now what happens? Some men admire me, but I'm not interested in a man's admiration. I want to love and be loved. I'm sick of being admired, if you really want to know – of Roberto's admiration and of yours. I regret having faked myself. How would I be if I hadn't gone against my essence? I faked myself, put on a mask to satisfy you. I was stupid and I'm angry with you – I have a bone to pick with you! Now I'm old enough to hear the truth. I want you to tell me – eye to eye – the way that you taught me. I'm going to stare into your eyes and I want you to tell me what you really felt . . . I need the truth!

P/F: My daughter, I think that really loving you . . . I loved you one day before I died. It was so good to have had you with me that day . . .

T/P: On that day it was really love?

P/F: Yes, I even felt a little lighter . . .

T/P: It's true, that day something different happened between us.

The therapist ends the role-play of the patient and the patient the role-play of the father.

Videotape technique

T: Close your eyes a little. Visualize this last day with your father. Notice the look in his eyes. Visualize an energy leaving his eyes and enveloping your body. On this day it is really love. The energy runs through your body. You don't need to pretend anymore, you can be real. Visualize the color of this energy and also some music that accompanies this movement. [A few minutes pass.] Very slowly, return to this room. How do you feel? Let's rest a little. You've worked enough.

References

Bowlby, J. (1958). The nature of the child's tie to his mother. *International Journal of Psychoanalysis*, 39: 350–372.

Buber, M. (1977). *Eu e tu*. São Paulo: Cortez e Moraes. (English American edition: *I and thou*. New York: Charles Scribner's Sons, 1970.)

Bustos, D. M. (1979). *Psicoterapia psicodrámatica (Psychodramatic psychotherapy)*. São Paulo: Brasiliense.

Fiorini, H. J. (1978). *Teoria y técnica de psicoterapia (Theory and technique of psychotherapy)*. Buenos Aires: Nueva Visión.

Fonseca, J. (1980). *Psicodrama da loucura (The psychodrama of madness)*. São Paulo: Ágora.

Fonseca, J. (1996). Psicodrama interno (Internal psychodrama). *Leituras* 16: 1–6.

Freud, S. (1968). *Obras completas*. Madrid: Editorial Biblioteca Nueva. (English edition: *The standard edition of the complete psychological works*.)

Greenson, R. (1982). *Investigações em psicanálise*. Rio de Janeiro: Imago. (Original edition: *Explorations in psychoanalysis*. New York: International Universities Press, Inc., 1978.)

Laing, R. D. (1972). *A psiquiatria em questão*. Lisboa: Presença. (Original edition: *The politics of experience and the bird of paradise*. Harmondsworth: Penguin Books, 1967.)

Moreno, J. L. (1977). *Psychodrama – First Volume* (5th edn). New York: Beacon House, Inc.

Perls, F. S. (1976). *Gestalt-terapia explicada*. São Paulo: Summus. (Original edition: *Gestalt therapy verbatim*. New York: Bantam, 1969.)

Winnicott, D. W. (1975). *O brincar e a realidade*. Rio de Janeiro: Imago Editora Ltda. (Original edition: *Playing and reality*. London: Tavistock Publications Ltd, 1971.)

Chapter 6

Internal psychodrama

Working with internal images*

Internal psychodrama is another clinical technique created from the anguish of the psychodramatist confined to an individual psychotherapy setting. Deprived of auxiliary egos, the stage, and the group, what remains for the dramatization, beyond the patient, sole and constant protagonist, are the objects available in the room. Naturally, the emotional climate achieved differs from that in a group situation, but attempts to surpass this limit have been made. Some of these techniques are: bipersonal psychodrama (Bustos, 1975), psychogram (Altenfelder Silva Filho, 1981), psychodrama with toys (Kaufman, 1978), psychodrama with dolls (Guerra, 1980), and the use of play in psychodrama (Fonseca, 1973).

The psychodramatist, accustomed to the group action technique, feels psychodramatically paralyzed in individual psychotherapy, whether this is admitted or not. Psychodramatists frequently employ techniques which originate from other theories, since Moreno did not address this theme. This is only fitting since he preferred psychotherapy in open groups to individual psychotherapy, which is private and "confessional" as he said.

Internal psychodrama is one technique I have employed in individual psychotherapy, and, depending on the circumstances, even in group psychotherapy.

The first time I heard of work with internal images was in the 1970s when A. C. M. Godoy, a Brazilian psychodramatist and bioenergist, told me that he achieved dramatizations with the client imagining the scenes. I found this interesting, but my impression was that the technique would not create a sufficiently emotional therapeutic level. However, I also watched Dalmiro Bustos realizing classical psychodramatic scenes in which he requested the protagonist to close his/her eyes and visualize a scene that Bustos would then stage. Later, Victor Silva Dias reported on what, at that time, he called

---

* Paper originally presented in the Second Brazilian Congress of Psychodrama, Canela, Rio Grande do Sul, 1980. It has been modified for the present publication.

mental psychodrama. The spontaneous way that internal images flowed from the patients called my attention. Following this, Silva Dias and I elaborated our own form of working with internal visual images. We have presented this technique in various public demonstrations during professional events, including the Second Brazilian Congress of Psychodrama in 1980.

I have had some personal experiences that were important in developing this technique – in particular the relaxation sessions that I did with the physical therapist Dorothea Hanser, in which, along with the corporeal manipulation, she suggested that the patient visualize his/her internal organs, had a significant influence. Other techniques from Gestalt therapy and bioenergetics were also valuable. Bioenergetics via body exercises (which work psychodramatically as a physical warm-up) provoke second states of consciousness from which internal images are generated. Once, in a workshop directed by Gerda Boyesen, one of the participants began to re-live experiences from her past after performing some specific exercises. With her eyes closed, she saw a scene from her childhood in which she talked with her mother. Gerda said, "What is your mother saying? How did you respond?" The protagonist experienced and narrated the episode. At that moment, it was clear to me that one could say: "You are the mother", or assume an internal role reversal. I came to believe that, in this manner, a psychodramatic resolution to conflict could be attempted.

During the initial development of the techniques in question, I employed body exercises suggested by a variety of different corporeal psychotherapeutic approaches. After working with muscle tension (increase and discharge of tension, seeking relaxation), I reached the moment in which visual images began to bud. As time passed, however, and as I gained intimacy with the procedure, I began to realize that this type of warm-up was unnecessary. Currently, I ask the patient to close his/her eyes and become conscious of the sensations present in his/her body at that moment. This process is frequently done with the patient lying down, but can also be effective with the patient seated, as long as he/she is comfortable and it is possible to relax the muscles. I ask the patient not to pay attention to thoughts, but to focus his/her attention on body sensations. Frequently I say: "Don't fight with, nor feed, your thoughts. Let them come and go freely, as if 'in one ear and out the other'. Put your attention on the body sensations present at this moment. Travel through your body, beginning with the head, and go along, registering the sensations." After remaining still with eyes closed for some time, the patient reports more significant sensations. I accompany this series of images as they develop spontaneously. By increasing body consciousness and decreasing the flow of thoughts, the process of internal image visualization is initiated. These images can appear through colors, shapes, movements, objects, scenes (landscapes), human figures, and unknown or past scenes.

The English psychiatrist Maurice Nicoll's statement (1980) that we function with seven vital regulating "centers"[1] – the emotional center, the intellectual center, the instinctive center, the motor center, the sexual center, the superior emotional center and the superior intellectual center – is important in understanding *internal psychodrama*. As the name itself elucidates, the emotional center is the regulator of emotions, sensations and feelings. The intellectual center coordinates thought. The instinctive center takes charge of the autonomous functioning of the internal organs. The motor center is responsible for coordinating movements generated by the muscles. The sexual center commands the sexual aspects of life in a broad sense. The two superior centers (the superior emotional center and the superior intellectual center) correspond to human functioning in a special sphere of life. Normally, they are activated in suitable and specific situations. They are the centers of human wisdom. For some theorists (like Jung, for example), they correspond to the *old wise man* that we all have within us. The superior emotional center can be manifested through premonitions, revelations and visions, such as those described by the prophets in the Bible. The superior emotional center is eminently visual. The superior intellectual center can reveal itself, for example, when a scientist, upon awakening, has a spontaneous resolution to a problem that bothered him for a long time. However, for most people, both centers are activated only in special situations.

These seven centers can, in a didactic sense, be consolidated into three centers: the *emotional center* (emotional center plus superior emotional center), the *intellectual center* (intellectual center plus superior intellectual center), and the *instinctive-motor center* (instinctive center plus motor center plus sexual center). Each center possesses its own language. This being so, the language of the emotional center is visual. Memories charged with feeling flow visually (I remember that situation as if it were yesterday!). When death is imminent, a person frequently visualizes scenes from the past. The language of the intellectual center is eminently verbal and manifests itself through words. But, certainly, determined words also have a visual appeal. Thus, I believe that thought has a secondary visual component that is distinguished from the visual described as a characteristic of the emotional center. In other words, the visual component of the emotional center is clearer, more defined and colored. It is three-dimensional in a way that the visual component of the intellectual center is not. The instinctive-motor center manifests itself through movement, whether movement of the internal organs, or the movement and balance involved in external body action.

---

1 Here the word "center" refers to function rather than anatomy, as each of the centers receives stimuli originating from various parts of the nervous system.

A complex chain of proprioceptive and exteroceptive sensors participates in this dynamic. In short, the language of the emotional center is visual; the language of the intellectual center is thought expressed verbally (with a secondary visual component); and the language of the instinctive-motor center is movement. The three centers are interconnected in their functioning by way of neurological and biochemical structures. Health depends on the harmony of the three centers. Imbalance in one of the centers will be reflected immediately in the other two. One could imagine the three centers as pulleys in a machine. If one of the pulleys rotates at a greater speed than the others it will rob energy from the system, resulting in disequilibrium. For example, if the intellectual center pulley were rotating much faster than normal it would consume an enormous amount of energy; then, the emotional and instinctive-motor centers would be harmed and begin to emit signals. From a medical point of view we would have a person with specific symptoms of psychosomatic disequilibrium.

The emotional center is difficult to observe directly. Often, a person becomes emotionally negative without noticing. Dominating the emotional center is difficult. It is not enough that the individual wants to not be sad, for example. If a person is depressed, it is useless for a friend to say, "Cheer up; life is beautiful and the sky is blue." Yet the intellectual and instinctive-motor centers are slower, facilitating self-observation. Thus, if I maintain a favorable posture, I can observe my body and determine its level of tension–relaxation. If I pay attention, I can verify the flow of thoughts that cross my consciousness at any given moment. If I prolong this exercise of attention–concentration, I will be able to reach a state that is a *window* to the emotional center; in other words, I can perceive my feelings and emotions with more acuity. They may be revealed directly or through visual images.

With this technique, one calms the intellectual and motor centers, so that the emotional center can appear more clearly through internal visual images.

Internal psychodrama is correlated with oriental meditation techniques. Both work in the sphere of *non-thought*. The analogy of a train in movement may clarify: the train would be the human mind and the cars would be the thoughts. We can focus our attention on the cars (thoughts) that pass by, in the way that psychoanalysis proposes the *association of ideas*. We can also observe the *gap* between the wagons, another form of observing the human mind. Meditation techniques and *internal psychodrama* utilize this approach.

There is some confusion when we speak of visualization. Many people mistake it for daydreams (automatic imagination of the daily life). Upon closer scrutiny, however, we see that they are opposites. The most significant difference is that visualization is reached by concentration and deliberate attention; in other words, there is a conscious effort to obtain it.

A daydream is the fruit of dispersion, of distraction, of non-attention. In visualization, the "practicer" dominates the process, is active in it. While daydreaming, the subject is passive, hence dominated. In visualization, the subject "rides" the experience, while in daydreaming the subject "is ridden". Tulku (1984) found that these quality differences are reflected in the type of visual images encountered. In visualizations, the images are intense, clear and three-dimensional, while daydreams have a poor variety of color, shapes and sounds. Visualizations result from a more profoundly altered state of consciousness; daydreams are superficial and dense. This does not mean that daydreams cannot have psychological or psychopatho-logical importance, even though they can be categorized as mental automatisms.[2]

Visualization takes place in a different state of consciousness. Between sleep and wakefulness there are various states of consciousness that corre-spond to different "knowledges" (infinite truths) of ourselves. Nicoll (1980) speaks of four states of human consciousness. The first, nocturnal sleep, is how we spend one-third of our lives. The second state is how we spend the rest of our lives: we walk, we talk, we love, we participate in politics, and we kill each other. This is the so-called "vigilant state". The third state is the consciousness, perception, or memory of oneself. Only by paying attention to oneself can one begin to develop this third state. Here, true "awakening" begins. Therefore, we can say that humans in the first two states of consciousness are "asleep" and only begin to truly awaken in the third. The first two states represent *darkness*; the third and fourth, *light*. The fourth state of consciousness, *illumination*, is difficult to describe as it transcends words. This state has been studied more by religions than by traditional science. Nevertheless, modern psychology has begun to concern itself with manifestations of this type.

Internal psychodrama can be viewed as an exercise in paying attention to oneself (like in meditative practices) and, thus, as practice for the third state of consciousness. The word *attention*, employed many times in this text, does not refer to mechanic attention, attracted automatically to external stimuli, but rather to attention deliberately directed. This is the attention utilized by an individual doing *internal psychodrama*, assisted by the psychotherapist. Daydreams, as I have already said, would be considered mechanic attention.

In this sense, I suggest that patients let their "internal film" flow, or that they begin to see with their "inner eye". I accompany them through what they relate to me; I see vicariously through them. The patient is my guide

---

2 Mental automatisms can be defined as being part of the independent functioning of the psychic life, the edge of dominating the will, and, sometimes, the consciousness. There are normal and pathological automatisms. For further information, see Porot (1967).

and I follow. It is common for patients to state that they perceive me as a voice from outside. I used to believe that the main point of internal psychodrama was the resolution of conflicts; today, I think that free, internal traveling or the flowing of spontaneity is most important. I believe in the human capacity for self-resolution or self-cure. Sometimes I employ psychodramatic techniques and other times cinematographic techniques. In this way, I maximize sensations, soliloquies, *role reversals* with human figures or objects and mirrors (I ask the patient to look from outside the scene and see him/herself in the situation). I suggest "close-ups", "zooms" and "panoramas" of these scenes. I think it is important for people to be aware that they are capable of creating – that we are all potential artists capable of producing impressive works, even if they are short-lived, as Moreno taught us.

When I started using *internal psychodrama*, I encouraged the motor release of emotional tensions in bioenergetics: kicking, biting, screaming, etc. Today, I ask the patient to look at, to verify in (his/her) *internal film*, the corresponding vision of tension discharges, while keeping the body still. The cinematographic techniques of *internal psychodrama* are more refined than the theatrical techniques of classical psychodrama. For example, the aggressive discharges in *internal psychodrama* add (thanks to the flexibility of the cinematographic technique), a variety of possibilities such as beating up a bully, destroying houses, disfiguring faces, etc. At other times during *internal psychodrama*, the use of color enriches the scene. I frequently suggest that a situation be visualized with the color corresponding to the protagonist's feeling.

While this technique may not be novel, it does involve a specific form of working with internal visual images (visualizations). Sandor (1974) states that internal images, as in dreams, are of vital necessity and he demonstrates how the image phase occurs in the catatonic process (by touching the feet which produces relaxation and the appearance of images that could, afterward, be worked through with the psychotherapist). Jung (1954) uses the term *active imagination*. Desoille (1973) denominates his method "guided daydream". He suggests the theme to be visualized by the client. Assagioli (1980) presents similar techniques. In Brazil, Hossri (1974) presents the "guided daydream" based on the methods of Schultz (self-training) and Desoille. I have not found concomitant working of the images among these methods (with the exception of Ericksonian hypnosis). In general, the images are produced to be elaborated on later.

When I have a dream, I, and only I, produce it – it is an exclusive work. We are natural dramaturges and directors. Hallucinations have the same characteristics. The visual images that come up in internal psychodrama are related to those of dreams and hallucinations and are, therefore, of profound origin. Dreams and visual images are vital necessities to humans. Hallucinations are the violent and uncontrolled eruption of something repressed. This abrupt manifestation signifies a desperate attempt to obtain mental re-equilibrium.

In *The interpretation of dreams*, Freud (1988) writes that dreams and daydreams have similar structures (manifest content and latent thoughts), subject to interpretation, therefore, by the same technical rules. I believe this is also applicable to visualizations. However, the methodology of *internal psychodrama* is opposite to that of psychoanalysis; while the latter tries to decipher (analyze in parts to reach the hidden unconscious sense) dreams or daydreams, *internal psychodrama* (and classical psychodrama) proposes to continue visualizing (to dramatize) in search of the connection or gestaltic *comprehension* of the experience. In this sense, Moreno's words to Freud at their encounter in Vienna at the beginning of the century perfectly reflect the differences in these methods: "You analyze (persons') dreams, I try to give them courage to dream again." We may say that, in either method, *interpretation* exists, but with different meanings. Psycho-analysis seeks to interpret dreams, viewing their unconscious content. According to Freud, this unconscious content hides unrealized desires, which go back to childhood, and, despite exceptions to the contrary, always reveals sexual conflicts. In psychodrama, *interpretation*[3] occurs in the sense that the dramatization of the dream reveals its meaning to the dreamer.

In *internal psychodrama*, the image prevails over the word, or forms an image–word binomial where the image comes first, like in cinema. Garcia-Roza (1993, p. 61), commenting on the path of the image to word for Freud, says that, "the Freudian proposal, with the interpretation of dreams, is to work through the passing of images in the dream, related by the dreamer, to the text to be interpreted". For Freud, the image conceals, not reveals, the true desire. Garcia-Roza further comments that there is no communion between the Freudian proposal and that of cinema: "While cinema will build a true mystique of the image, Freud will elaborate his theory over the ruins of the image's temple (Lacoste)" (p. 61). Cinema and dream psychoanalysis point in opposite directions; the former puts symbolic discussion into images, while the latter passes image to word. In this sense, as we can see, *internal psychodrama* is more cinema than psychoanalysis.

Internal psychodrama does not insist that the image be concealing. As I have already commented, the registering and evoking of visual images is the result of the emotional center, just as verbal expression runs from the intellectual center and action runs from the instinctive-motor center. With this approach, none of the three languages is inherently concealing but can

---

3 In respect to the *interpretation* in psychodrama, consult Wilson Castello de Almeida's paper "Interpretar e a função interpretativa da dramatização", presented in the 9th Brazilian Congress of Psychodrama, Águas de São Pedro, São Paulo, November 1994.

be, depending on the circumstances and the balance/imbalance of the three centers. For example, in classical psychodrama and in systematic family therapy, it is common to suggest that the protagonist should transform the verbal account into a *symbolic image* or *allegory*, or a *sculpture*. He/she then uses people and objects to translate the hidden contents of the verbal account into an image – either plastic, static, or in movement – followed by the role-play of these different parts. In this case, the concealing language would be verbal.

Internal psychodrama does not seek the resolution of conflicts exclusively, but, perhaps more importantly, tries to discover and calibrate channels of expression, essential for communication between the conscious and unconscious.

I use *internal psychodrama* in a more orthodox form, beginning with only the body sensations present at the moment, with no preconceived idea (the patient's or mine) or specific question to be approached – a real trip into the unknown – navigating by the body sensations and visualizations which come up. At other times I employ visualizations in work with dreams or in situations that have occurred. In these cases, when re-visualizing a scene, we work with the emotional impact of the moment, "presentifying" the past. I also use visualization flashes in classical psychodramatic scenes. In these last examples, I prefer to use the term *videotape technique*, which is, in effect, a derivation of *internal psychodrama*. This technique utilizes immediate visualizations of significant scenes from the patient's dreams or real life. I have observed that closed-eyed visualization helps to avoid already intellectualized evocative memory ("semantic memory" as we will see ahead). In these moments, I ask the patients to focus their attention on body sensations and simply look within themselves.

Some people manage internal dramatization with much greater ease than in classical form. *Role reversal* also becomes easier in *internal psychodrama*. In classical psychodrama, movement is necessary for the dramatization. It is entirely different to attack a person physically in the "as if" of a classic psychodrama scene than to attack with all of the refinement of imagination. The corporeal act in classical psychodrama can sometimes lift insurmountable phobic barriers. Moreno (1977) claims that the child plays the role of another at the fantasy level before playing the role at the level of playful representation. For example, as a child, I would imagine that I am a doctor, and what it is like to be a doctor; later, I would propose playing a doctor, but in order to do so I would need companions that represent the roles of the patient, nurse, etc. Therefore, while playing the role at the level of imagination is, on the one hand, a natural process of development, it could also be, in certain situations, a way of avoiding interacting with the others who play complementary roles. We observe that the same process occurs in adults. Imaginary roles function as training for action. For example, if I am going to speak to a very important person I do a mental role-play of the

situation; afterward, I go to speak to "Mr. Intimidating". But if my fear/
inhibition continues, I will not go to speak with him in reality; I will
continue inventing countless images. In the refuge of myself, where I am
alone and no one can see me, I am a hero, bandit, poet and king. Here I
play roles without the interference of external resistance. *Internal psychodrama* encompasses this internal role-playing. As mentioned in Chapter 1, I
define *pre-reversal*, or *role-playing the other*, as a development phase. This
should be further subdivided into two stages: role-play at the level of the
imagination (internal view) and at the level of action. Two types of fantasy
will result from this: *fantasy-imagination* and *fantasy-action*. I have also
already asserted that a psychotic has difficulty in, or is entirely incapable of,
reversing roles in classic psychodrama. Based on the above discussion, it
would be expected that in *internal psychodrama* he/she would demonstrate
more ease – which is what has been observed. A psychotic is more comfortable with *internal psychodrama* than in the classical form. He/she will be
more blocked for fantasy action but less so for fantasy imagination.
However, the therapist must establish sufficient trust to be able to employ
internal psychodrama in psychotics, as with any client, for that matter.

Since scenes from the past do occasionally occur in *internal psychodrama*,
a word or two on memory is appropriate. I take the same position as
Bowlby (1981) and Nicoll (1980). Summarizing Bowlby, there are two
memories: *semantic memory* and *episodic memory*. *Semantic memory* is
the register of episodes according to the emotional needs at the moment
of occurrence and (I believe) of the emotional necessities at the moment of
recollection. This memory, frequently neurotic, then serves to defend the
ego. For Nicoll, this would be a mechanized and repetitive memory filtered
only by the intellectual center. According to Bowlby, the second type of
memory, *episodic memory*, has hidden emotional meaning, which contains
imprisoned affective energy awaiting liberation. For Nicoll, this *new
memory*, a full memory, would correspond to the memory of the three
centers (intellectual, emotional and instinctive-motor), functioning harmoniously among themselves. To obtain this second (true) memory, we
need to revert and psychodramatically recreate the original situation,
returning to experience the forgotten parts of the episodes. It is as if we
need to return to the place where something was forgotten to be able to
bring it back home with us. It is like a movie scene filmed by three cameras
(or from three standpoints), but which reveals only one angle on film. We
must salvage the *takes* obtained by the two other cameras to gain a new,
more complete comprehension of the global story.

Example

The *internal psychodrama* session described here shows the first stage of my
work with internal images, in which classical psychodramatic and

bioenergetic techniques were mixed with some frequency. This session, which addresses an issue that came up during the patient's work in group therapy, was chosen for its didactic quality in exposing the technique. I have left out the occasional psychodynamic comment in order to highlight the presentation of the technique.

1   During the group psychotherapy session there were a series of verbal confrontations in which one of the participants referred to this patient as a boring, awkward, humorless man. This scene persists within him, so I decide to interrupt the group work to conduct this session of internal psychodrama. Shortly after lying down and closing his eyes the patient identifies a heavy sensation in his chest and proceeds to visualize the scene, which occurred in the group.

2   I ask the patient to concentrate on the feeling in his chest, to immerse himself in it, and to follow along with the internal vision. He immediately sees a scene from his adolescence. His mother admonishes him after discovering a girl's telephone number in his pocket. She warns him that if he continues entangling himself with women at such a young age he will amount to nothing in life. His father, watching, supports his mother.

3   Again, a heavy sensation in his chest leads him to another scene. He is younger, still a boy. The family is together for a celebration. His mother exclaims: "Let's attack", referring, symbolically, to getting lunch started. The boy takes her comment literally and *attacks* the food, getting ahead of the others. He receives a tremendous reprimand from his father, who calls him "awkward" and sends him from the table.

4   The bodily concretization of these feelings is perceived as an impact that produces a *hole in his stomach*. I ask him to pay attention to the hole. He begins to feel tremors that leave this hole and descend to his feet. There are waves, some of which leave through his feet while others do not. I suggest that he follow the tremors, not fight against them.

5   The tremors increase in intensity. His whole body trembles. He is consumed by the tremors.

6   After a few minutes, the tremors diminish. The protagonist calms down a little. He then visualizes darkness with small twinkling points in movement. "It seems like the cosmos." Little by little, a center opens up. I ask that he get closer, if he feels like it, and penetrate this center or hole.

7   A scene from his childhood comes up in which, being very small and light-skinned, he is mocked by three young adults. He identifies the three. They make jokes that he doesn't understand well: "A guy who kills crows goes to prison", as if he killed crows. One of them shows a sexual interest in the boy's mother, another, for the boy himself. He is

terrified, full of fear. I ask him to pay attention, to become physically aware of his fear.

8   The physical sensation of the fear causes him to start to float and grow. His body feels enormous. "I'm turning into a giant, an enormous sensation of power and force." I encourage him: "OK, let's go on."

9   His penis grows as if it was a huge palm tree, bends and urinates on one of the aggressors. "A wonderful feeling. I wouldn't kill him, but a voice says to kill him, so I twist his neck."

10 At this time, he is overwhelmed by feelings of well-being and that his body is swinging sideways. The movement grows until he starts to rotate. "I was completely dizzy. I lost my sense of space." I then suggest that, with his eyes closed, he get up and make a rotating movement with his body.[4]

11 "A sensation of having entered through the window. As if something is pulling me to the floor. I turned and turned, and when I fell I heard the sound of all my bones. It was a fearless fall. I started to breathe deeply. Then came a hiccup and convulsive crying, a feeling of abandonment. A terrible feeling leaving through crying and exhaling. Then came a feeling of well-being, of happiness. Maybe you could have helped physically, on the chest, as one does with a baby."[5]

12 A feeling of coziness, protection and peace follows. A new scene: "I must be about four years old. I'm looking through the window of the house. It's raining outside; my mother is sewing; no one is talking. The house is hot. It's a feeling of wholeness."

13 The return: "A feeling of filling up space, of presence. It wasn't just a physical thing. It was something connected to me. I felt that I was in the whole space. I felt a great love for people and a great desire for physical contact. I have difficulty with physical contact, but what I gave and what I received was entirely spontaneous."

References

Altenfelder Silva Filho, L. M. (1981). Psicograma: utilização do desenho em psicoterapia psicodramática (Psychograma: utilization of design in psychodramatic psychotherapy). *Temas*, 21: 101–127.

Assagioli, R. (1980). *Psychosynthesis*. New York: Penguin Books.

4 Later, the patient commented that he was irritated with my suggestion and his realization, "The physical movement took away a harmonious movement that was moving toward something I don't know." After comments such as this, I stopped physically mobilizing the protagonist during the session and allowed the action to elapse through internal visualizations only.

5 At this point, the patient shows the importance of physical contact to opportune moments in the session.

Bowlby, J. (1981). *Loss: sadness and depression.* Vol. III: *Attachment and loss.* New York: Penguin Books.

Bustos, D. M. (1975). *Psicoterapia psicodramática (Psychodramatic psychotherapy).* Buenos Aires: Paidós.

Castello de Almeida, W. (1994). Interpretar e a função interpretativa da dramatização (Interpreting and the interpretive function of dramatization). IX Congresso Brasileiro de Psicodrama, Águas de São Pedro, São Paulo.

Desoille, R. (1973). *Entretiens sur le rêve éveillé dirigé en psychothérapie* (Commentaries on evoked dreams directed in psychotherapy). Paris: Payot.

Fonseca, J. (1973). O uso de elementos lúdicos em psicodrama (The use of play in psychodrama). Sociedade de Psicodrama de São Paulo, São Paulo.

Fonseca, J. (1980). *Psicodrama da loucura (The psychodrama of madness).* São Paulo: Ágora.

Freud, S. (1970–1977). *Projeto para uma psicologia científica (1895–1950).* ESB. Vol. I. Edição Brasileira das Obras Psicológicas Completas de Sigmund Freud, Rio de Janeiro: Imago. (English edition: *A project for a scientific psychology.* The standard edition of the complete works of Sigmund Freud, vol. 1. London: Hogarth Press, 1954.)

Freud, S. (1988). *A interpretação dos sonhos.* Rio de Janeiro: Imago. (English edition: *The interpretation of dreams.* Standard edition, vols 4–5, 1900.)

Garcia-Roza, L. A. (1993). *Introdução à metapsicologia freudiana (Introduction to Freudian metapsychology).* Rio de Janeiro: Zahar.

Guerra, F. A. (1980). Em busca de uma linguagem comum (In search of a common language). II Congresso Brasileiro de Psicodrama, Canela, RS.

Hossri, C. M. (1974). *Sonho acordado dirigido. Onirodrama de grupo (Guided daydream. Group dream-drama).* São Paulo: Mestre Jou.

Jung, C. G. (1954). *The collected works of C. G. Jung.* London: Routledge & Kegan Paul.

Kaufman, A. (1978). O jogo em psicoterapia individual (The game in individual psychotherapy). *Revista da FEBRAP,* 1, 2: 82–86.

Moreno, J. L. (1977). *Psychodrama – First Volume* (5th edn). New York: Beacon House, Inc.

Nicoll, M. (1980). *Comentários psicológicos sobre las enseñanzas de Gurdjieff y Ouspensky.* Buenos Aires: Kier. (Original edition: *Psychological commentaries on the teaching of Gurdjieff and Ouspensky.* London: Vincent Stuart Publishers, 1952.)

Porot, A. (1967). *Dicionário de psiquiatria (Psychiatric dictionary).* Barcelona: Labor.

Sandor, P. (1974). *Técnicas de relaxamento (Relaxation techniques).* São Paulo: Vetor.

Tulku, T. (1984). *Gestos de equilíbrio.* São Paulo: Pensamento. (Original edition: *Gesture of balance: a guide to awareness, self-healing and meditation.* Berkeley, CA: Dharma Publishing, 1977.)

Chapter 7

The patient, the illness and the body
A view through internal psychodrama*

I receive a patient who has been sent by a cardiologist. He is a 51-year-old man, financially accomplished, married, with two adult children. He presents a coronary circulatory deficiency and is recommended for surgery. In addition to chest pain he presents an "exaggerated" psychological reaction, according to his physician. Upon receiving the diagnosis, he became depressed, suffered bouts of crying and assumed a pessimistic attitude toward the results of the treatment. He was directed to a psychiatrist in the hopes of improving his psychological condition for the surgery. I've chosen the second session, of three held in one week, related here in abbreviated form.

The session begins with the patient lying down. I ask him to get comfortable, close his eyes and refrain from moving until the end of the session. I suggest that he pay attention to his bodily sensations and that he ignore whatever thoughts he may have. In the following, I report the primary moments of the *internal psychodrama* carried out:

1   The predominant feeling is a light weight on the chest.
2   He concentrates on this region and delineates the sensation as the form of an egg, approximately 20 by 30 cm.
3   He visualizes the color of the egg as grey.
4   Focusing on the grey egg, he reports that it has become a grey rock.
5   The rock grows. I suggest that he watch the scene from outside (*internal mirror technique*). He sees himself with the rock on his chest. The *mirror technique* permits the protective distance necessary for the next scene.
6   The rock grows enormously and the visualized patient in the scene bursts like an inflatable rubber doll. The patient, observing, is stupefied.

* Work presented at the Second International Congress on the Body, Rio de Janeiro, May, 1987, and at the Twenty-fifth Anniversary Congress on Psychodrama in Buenos Aires, Argentina, August, 1988. Published in *Revista Brasileira de Psicodrama*, vol. 2, fac. 1, pp. 41–48, 1994.

7   He feels dizzy. He reports feeling a sensation of wind blowing against him.

8   Attentive to the wind, he sees himself walking along a street with many pedestrians. He identifies it as Direita Street, in downtown São Paulo. He is wearing clothing from the 1940s. He wears a suit and hat and is very thin. (In the 1940s, the patient was a boy, but in the scene he is an adult.)

9   Putting his attention on the act of walking, he is transported to a desert. He is walking, completely alone. He is wearing a hat with a wide brim. He stresses the unpleasant sensation of loneliness. I ask him to observe this sensation, which is the point of the visualization of the next scene.

10   He visualizes himself as a boy, apparently five years old. Night is falling; it is cold. He is in his hometown. He is lost and cannot find his house. He is afraid and cries. He has become separated from his older brother with whom he had gone to an amusement park. He longs for his mother and his home.

11   I suggest that he look at the boy (*mirror technique*) and watch the scene unfold as if it were a dream.

12   He is crying and calling for his mother. His *physical body* (in the session) presents light tremors and he has tears in his eyes. He finally finds his house. He runs in through the gate and throws himself into his mother's arms; she lovingly receives him.

13   He feels his mother's warmth and smell. He experiences a sensation of fullness.

14   He feels his body tingling and relaxed. I ask him to visualize the color of the tingling. After a brief silence, he states that the color is bright pink. I suggest that he follow the bright pink color spreading over his body.

15   I start the process of returning, indicating that when his whole body has been filled with the bright pink color, that he return to the room where we are and observe (*internal visualization*) the sensation of his adult body with the same color. I also ask him to look at his colored body from above (*mirror*) and that he "savor" the image.

16   Little by little, he returns to a normal state of consciousness, moving and opening his eyes. He feels good.

We talk about the sensations he experienced. In the next session we comment on and analyze the material from the previous session. He informs me that he has set up a date for the surgery. He is apprehensive but confident. He makes plans to change the pace of his professional life and "take more advantage of life". I begin to weave a few theoretical reflections from the case.

Autotele and autotransference

Firstly, re-living the past is not only connected to *transferential* processes but also to *telic* processes. The patient displays an inappropriate reaction toward his illness. I presume that the lost boy of the past represents the frightened adult of the present and that the patient was indiscriminately repeating the past and distorting the circumstantial reality of the present. On the other hand, it was also through the past that he salvaged positive energy – *telic* – in the sense of re-establishing homeostatic balance.

Along these lines, it is necessary to understand the concept of *autotele*, of which Moreno speaks so briefly in his work, and, by extension, the concept of *auto transference*, which I propose here.

Moreno (1966) refers to autotele when he discusses "the social atom of a psychotic world":

> As we have shown, in a normal social atom, an individual always has, besides the relationships based on the tele with others, a relationship with himself or "autotele" which is substituted in the sociogram of a psychotic by multiple roles. The original "autotele" then explodes into numerous fragments . . .
>
> (Moreno, 1966, pp. 346–347)

I understand, then, that the "exploded *autotele*", as Moreno says, is substituted for something that could coherently be called *auto transference*. This concerns an *autotele–autotransference process* in which man permanently oscillates. This process measures the perception, capture or consciousness of his/her own self; that is, the relationship of the individual with him/herself (*I–I*).[1] This is inserted in the *fantasy–reality* sphere because we are never exactly what we imagine ourselves to be. The *self-image* which oscillates between the (auto)*telic* and the (auto)*transferential* contains an external and internal corporeal aspect. The internal aspect refers to the internal organs – unseen, but felt in some way. The external aspect regards our aesthetic apprehension of ourselves. As health is classically described as a state of *organ silence*, illness would be *the noise of the organs*. In this patient's case, the heart begins to make *noise*. He initially reacts with autotransference. He feels lost and abandoned. The clinical reality in itself is worrisome, but becomes even graver when an autotransferential reaction comes up. He deposits his sensation of loneliness and desperation in the heart (the symbol of feeling).

---

1 The question of *autotele–autotransference* is incorporated in the larger chapter on teletransference. My concepts on the *teletransference* system can be consulted in *Psychodrama or neo-psychodrama?* (Fonseca, 1992).

The other bipolarity, besides the *teletransference* and *autotele-autotransference*, is that referring to *life–death*. This is the same bipolarity that measures *health–illness*. The intrinsic structure of both is *relationship–separation*, the basic existential element from the moment we arrive in the world until we depart from it. The human being oscillates between gestation (relationship) to birth (separation), between maternal caretaking (relationship) and the renouncement of it (separation), between love (relationship) and rejection (separation). Being ill sensitizes the consciousness of *life–death* and, therefore, of *relationship–separation*. The patient fears death-abandonment–separation, and desires life–health–relationship. Upon receiving a dose of relationship (mother)–life–health, the process is re-balanced.

The physical, psychological (symbolic), energetic body

At this time, we can make a distinction between the *physical body* and the *symbolic* or *psychological body*. The patient's *physical body* was ill. The *psychological* or *symbolic body* contained an underlying, latent, affective world, which the illness caused to emerge. The *psychological* or *symbolic* body is represented in this case by all the bodies the patient assumed during the internal psychodrama, especially the body of the lost boy in search of his mother. Before the surgical intervention on the *physical body*, we intervened in the *symbolic* or *psychological body*.

The interaction between the *physical* and the *symbolic bodies* results in a third: the *energetic body*. The greater the spontaneous fluency between the *physical* and *symbolic bodies*, the more harmonious the *energetic body* will be. The obstruction of spontaneous fluency would generate an overloaded *energetic body*, if it were possible to measure its energetic potential. I believe that greater understanding of the energetic body would be useful in that it could then be altered even before an illness manifests itself officially.

Internal images

Internal psychodrama acts as a *psychological surgery* and the warm-up process as *anesthesia*. The warm-up makes possible a state of consciousness favorable to internal images. In this case, the warm-up comprised the conscious and deliberate *attention* to the body, the reduction in the flow of thoughts, physical immobility and muscular relaxation.

The process of internal visual images was set off by Freud. He correlates them to dreams. According to Greenson (1982), internal images constitute a primitive process and are, therefore, closer to unconscious processes than verbal representation. I cite a passage from this author:

Even after the acquisition of speech, the thinking of a child is, essentially, dominated by pictorial representations . . . There are more primitive stampings which are derived from bodily states and infantile feelings which cannot be recorded, but which can give origin to mental images and sensations in dreams.

(Greenson, 1982, pp. 425–427)

I add: which can give rise to visual images in internal psychodrama. Just as the "dream is, essentially, a visual experience, the majority of adult recollections of early childhood come to us in the form of scenes or pictures" (Greenson, 1982, p. 426). The internal visual images of *internal psychodrama* are relatives of the dream and constitute a window for conscious–unconscious memory. Taking Greenson's (1982) idea that "the dream is the freest of free associations" (p. 426), one step further, I suggest that the internal images of internal psychodrama, after the dream, are the freest of free associations. The field of free association would have to be divided into the free association of ideas and that of images, which I judge to be substantially different processes. But moving into this territory must await another opportunity.

As a final note on the visualization of internal images, I don't worry about the significance of colors. Nor do I follow any explanatory code that correlates color to emotion. I propose to myself, as well as to others, to be a facilitator and amplifier of the phenomena that occur during the procedure. In this patient's case two colors appear – grey and bright pink – which, in themselves, speak of the bipolarities cited (illness–health, death–life, separation–relationship). Beyond this, I dare not go.

References

Fonseca, J. (1992). Psicodrama ou neo-psicodrama? (Psychodrama or neo-psychodrama?). *Psicodrama, Revista da SOPSP*, 4: 7–19.

Fonseca, J. (1994). O doente, a doença e o corpo. Visão através do psicodrama interno (The ill person, the illness and the body. A view through internal psychodrama). *Revista Brasileira de Psicodrama*, 2, 1: 41–48.

Greenson, R. R. (1982). *Investigações em psicanálise*. Rio de Janeiro: Imago. (Original edition: *Explorations in psychoanalysis*. New York: International Universities Press, Inc., 1978.)

Moreno, J. L. (1966). *Psicoterapia de grupo y psicodrama (Group psychotherapy and psychodrama)*. México City: Fondo de Cultura Económica. (Original edition: *Gruppenpsychotherapie und psychodrama. Einleitung in die theorie und praxis*. Stuttgart: Georg Thieme Verlag, 1959.)

Chapter 8

Theater psychodrama

Theater psychodrama is an experiment that combines traditional or "legitimate" theater, as Moreno said, with spontaneous theater or, in a broader sense, psychodrama. In Act I, corresponding to classical theater, a 40–50-minute play is presented. In Act II, a psychodramatic director warms up the audience to re-enact scenes from the play. The protagonists are people from the audience, while the actors from Act I become the auxiliary egos. Any scenes can be chosen and spontaneously transformed, according to the protagonists' emotions.

Freud, Moreno and Dora
Historical fiction
(Vienna, 1900–1915)
A play in two acts

Characters:
Dora, Father, Mother, Freud, Mrs K, Mr K, Moreno

Potential characters:
Governess, Brother, Fliess, and all that are created in Act II

Act I (theater)

Scene 1

[*Open space. Supposedly in the living room. The parents are seated; Dora is standing.*]

DORA: [*Walking nervously.*] I've said it before and I'll say it again: you have to fire that disgusting governess. And the K couple must never step foot in this house again. [*Cough, cough.*] They are despicable! [*She coughs and then, with a mixture of sarcasm, aggressiveness and malice, says:*] As for her, Mrs K, you know why, don't you, Dad . . .? [*A brief pause to observe her father's reaction, who withdraws a bit.*] And him, because he is repulsive, troublesome! [*Cough, cough. She starts breathing more and more heavily, falls to the floor, moans, contorts herself and makes convulsive–sensual movements. – A hysterical-convulsive fit. – The parents go to her and then help her leave the room.*]

Scene 2

[*Father and mother return to the room.*]

FATHER: I don't know what else to do . . .

MOTHER: [*Fragile appearance, a little "out of it", falling apart.*] Philip, I've already told you . . . She swears that Mr K tried to grab her again. She also said that you and Mrs K . . . Well, never mind . . . Have you spoken with Mr K?

FATHER: Yes, I have. He is a respectable man. I've known him for many years. He would be incapable of such a thing. He thinks, as do I, that she's been fantasizing excessively. She's been reading lewd books! She's been consumed with erotic daydreams. And you remember how, just a short time ago, she was infatuated with Mr and Mrs K? Now, she's become resentful and spends hours locked away in her room. Thinking or doing who-knows-what!

MOTHER: What makes me more worried is the note I found in her room saying that she'd kill herself. That she feels alone, abandoned . . . It's been two years since we were last at Dr Freud's office. Shouldn't we go to him again?

Scene 3

Dr. Freud's office

[*The stage is divided into three parts. In the middle is the office; flashback scenes occur on stage right; on the left is the communication between Freud and Fliess. When a scene takes place in one area, the other areas remain in half-light.*]

DORA: What's going on, Dr Freud, is that there is a family conspiracy. No one believes me. I may come off looking crazy, but the real crazy ones are those who act like nothing is happening.

FREUD: What is happening?

DORA: Mr and Mrs K are friends of my parents, I mean, of my father, because my mother is totally out of it.

FREUD: Out of it?

DORA: She doesn't take charge of anything. She's a fool. All she thinks about is picking up the house, washing and ironing. I think this is ridiculous. But men are, at the very least, accomplices to the plight of women. I don't think it's fair that men dominate women this way . . .

FREUD: [*Trying to calm her*] Well, well, well, Dora, let's get to the point!

FREUD: [*In soliloquy*] So young and already with these feminist ideas . . .

DORA: So, I was in love with them, with Mr and Mrs K.

FREUD: In love?

DORA: Yes, they were my idols. I thought that, when I grew up, I would be just like Mrs K and I wanted a husband just like Mr K. She seemed good, understanding. She was a friend. She spoke with me as if I were already grown up. And she was beautiful!

Scene 4

[*stage right*]

[*Mrs K is getting changed in front of an imaginary mirror. She opens her dress and closes it, in such a way that Dora can see her body*]

MRS K: How do I look?

DORA: You are beautiful. You have a wonderful body! Can I see it again? [Mrs K repeats the gesture]

[*Return to the office*]

FREUD: And now she's no longer beautiful?

DORA: Now I think she's a witch, horrible, disgusting, just like him.

FREUD: But how has such a radical transformation occurred? From excellent, they've become horrible!

DORA: Everything started when I was fourteen.

Scene 5

[*stage right*]

MR K: Dora, you're becoming a very beautiful woman!

DORA: Um, I'm not really a woman yet . . . It's your wife, Mrs K, who's beautiful.

MR K: You're prettier than she is. Just looking at you, I feel something strange! Come here Dora!

[*He grabs Dora, holds her against his body and kisses her on the lips. Dora is overwhelmed by the shock, but soon resists and manages to free herself from the embrace. She shows with a gesture – wiping her mouth with her hand – her repulsion*]

[*Return to the office*]

FREUD: But before the repulsion, what did you feel?

DORA: Just disgust, Dr Freud, just disgust. That wet mouth [*dubious*]. Oh, I can't forget . . .

FREUD: But, up until the time of the kiss, you liked him, admired him, loved him. It's easier to believe that you would have felt proud to have an older man desire you. The disgust hides the pleasure, the enjoyment that the moment brought you.

DORA: No, Dr Freud, no.

FREUD: I understand that you were in love with this attractive gentleman, although you denied to yourself your desire for him.

DORA: I don't think you understand me!

FREUD: But, and after that?

DORA: Later, I found out some things with the help of the governess. She's much older than I am, and experienced. She opened my eyes to some things. And I found out other things on my own.

FREUD: For example?

DORA: For example, that Mrs K has been my father's lover for a long time . . .

FREUD: But didn't you tell me in another session that your father is impotent?

DORA: But, Dr Freud, you know that there is more than just the "conventional" way of having sex!

FREUD: Are you suggesting that, let's put it this way, [*scratches his head*] that they practice oral sex?

[*Dora coughs several times as if in agreement*]

FREUD: [*in soliloquy*] But how can a girl, who only started her period a year ago, know such things?

DORA: [*As if she had heard*] I used to talk to the governess about sex. I don't talk with her any more because I found out that she, too, is in love with my father and was just using me to get information. Besides, I've read Mantegazza's book: The physiology of love.

FREUD: [*Surprised*] Mantegazza, Kraft-Ebing's disciple?

DORA: Exactly!

FREUD: [*More to himself than to her*] I don't believe it! [*Returning to the conversation*] But you said that the governess is "also" in love with your father. [*Suggesting that Dora is as well. He follows with a gesture indicating he's hit the nail on the head*]

DORA: She and Mrs K, Dr Freud! You are trying to insinuate that I'm
          in love with my father. I read an interview in the newspaper
          where you talk about daughters' passion for their fathers. But
          this is not my case, no. Did you know that there are people who
          think you're a little over the top about these things?

FREUD: Sure, you said that you don't feel a physical attraction for your
          father, but you could feel this for a substitute – Mr K.

DORA: Gee, you're going to start everything all over again! Dr Freud, he
          is an undignified man. I don't admire him anymore. I want to fall
          in love with an honest man, who I can admire, feel proud of. He
          knows that my father is his wife's lover and accepts this for
          commercial benefit. And now they're trying to put me in the
          middle of this conspiracy. My father "doesn't believe" that Mr K
          is trying to seduce me and Mr K "doesn't believe" that his wife is
          my father's lover. They want to get me involved in this trading,
          this bargaining of women. They're all accomplices. I don't have
          any allies. I need you to believe in me.

FREUD: I won't say that this can't be true, but I'm interested in revealing
          another truth, the truth of your unconscious.

Scene 6

[stage left]

[Freud sits down and starts writing]

FREUD: Oh, my dear Fliess, it's so good to have someone to talk to! I
          recommend an internal Fliess for everyone, a big ear that listens
          to you as that guy [it seems like he's going to say "Lacan", but he
          doesn't] will say . . . Take a look at this girl: [he points to the side
          of the divan] a petite histerique. For three years she's suffered
          from a nervous cough, aphonia, hoarseness, sadness, unsocia-
          bility, taedium vitae. Now there are fainting spells, dismal
          thoughts, hostility and thoughts of death. Her father, the poor
          man, who I treated for syphilis a few years ago, confided in me
          that the girl is pressuring him to cut his ties with the K couple.
          But he said, "Dr Freud, I can't do this, since, in the first place, I
          believe the immoral insinuations against Mr K are a fantasy that
          my daughter has gotten stuck in her head. Furthermore, I'm
          connected to Mr K by ties of honorable friendship . . . But Dora,
          who inherited my stubbornness, is obstinate in her hatred for the
          Ks." My dear Fliess, you know what "hysterical rancor" is? You
          need to see that, beyond the homosexual elements – for example,
          "your wonderful body" is an expression more appropriate for a

lover than a rival – there appears to be what is known as "gynecophylia", a generalized love for women as well as an exaggerated interest in women's rights. She has been going to feminist talks! The cough and loss of voice, which can be traced back to a kind of baby's sucking, and the main issue concerning the conflicting thoughts, is the contrast between an inclination for men and an inclination for women. The mother is described by the father as terrible in bed and a carrier of the syndrome called "housewife psychosis" – disinterest toward the children, manic obsession with cleanliness, frigidity, and a total lack of insight toward herself. One time Mr K was in my office, accompanying Dora's father, during his treatment for syphilis. A very good-looking man! A handsome man, you see. The erotic interest of an attractive man like Mr K would have to arouse clear feelings of sexual excitement in an innocent, fourteen-year-old girl. Normally, she would give in to the sexual harassment; that is to say, deep down, deep down, she wants . . . And in the end, Fliess, according to my previous studies, I classify, without hesitation, anyone for whom sexual excitement provokes disgust as hysterical.

[*Returning to the office*]

DORA: I'm sorry, Dr Freud, but the smell of that cigar is really strong. I'm starting to feel queasy; it's a little nauseating.

FREUD: [*Turning toward his office*] Fliess, listen to this, now it's coming at me!! [*and picking up with Dora*] Sure, sure. [*He puts out the cigar*]

DORA: But, as I was saying, Dr Freud, I'm not the silly little girl I was before. A year ago, when I was already sixteen, Mr K and I were going out, I mean, we went for a walk . . . [*Dr Freud smiles and slaps his hand against his thigh with Dora's "Freudian slip"*]

Scene 7

[*stage right*]

MR K: You know, Dora, my marriage practically doesn't exist any more.

DORA: How's that?

MR K: You know, "not getting any", you understand, from my wife.

DORA: [*In soliloquy*] What a son-of-a-bitch, repeating to me the same come-on he used with the governess. Good thing she told me everything!

[*In this interim, Mr K, inebriated with desire, moves in, hugs and gropes Dora. He stutters a few random, unconnected words: "You're so hot", etc.*]
[*Dora slaps Mr K on the face and looks at him triumphantly*]

[*Returning to the office*]

DORA: Oh, Dr Freud, I really gave him what he had coming!

FREUD: [*Delighted*] It gave you a real thrill, didn't it?

DORA: Oh, it sure did – I cleaned my soul!

FREUD: You confirm my hypothesis. The pleasure of your aggression was just like an orgasm.

DORA: Spare me, Dr Freud. Is this the only thing you ever think about?

FREUD: [*A little disappointed*] Well, maybe we can work on a dream then . . . [*Proudly*] I'm good at this! I've just finished writing a book on dreams!

DORA: All right. I dreamed that there was a house in flames. My father, who was right next to my bed, woke me up. I got dressed quickly. My mother wanted to salvage her jewelry box, but my father said: "I refuse to burn to death, along with my two children, because of your jewelry box." We went down the stairs quickly and I woke up outside the house.

FREUD: What do you associate the jewelry box with?

DORA: Mr K gave me a box like that, an expensive present in fact!

FREUD: You know that "jewelry box" is an expression that alludes to the female genital organs?

DORA: I knew you were going to say that!

FREUD: This is it, *you know*. The meaning of your dream is becoming even clearer. You said to yourself: This man is after me; he even wants to get into my room. My "jewelry box" is in danger and, if something terrible happens, it will be my father's fault. It was because of this that you adopted a situation in your dream that expressed the opposite, a danger from which your father saves you. In this part of the dream, everything is converted to its opposite. Soon you'll know why. The secret certainly resides in your mother. How does your mother fit in here? She is, as you know, your old rival for your father's attention.
        [*Dora gestures with her hand, indicating that Freud is more or less on track*]

FREUD: In this way, you are willing to give as a gift what his wife has refused him. Here you have a thought that is repressed with such strength that it demands a conversion of all elements to their opposites. As I told you, the dream confirms that you are evoking the old love you nurture for your father, hoping to protect yourself from your love for Mr K. But what do all these efforts prove? Not only that you fear Mr K, but also that you fear yourself even more, the temptation to give in to him. [*He pauses and says triumphantly*] Our time is up.

[*Dora retreats, appearing tired, desolate. She shakes her head*]

FREUD: [*In soliloquy*] I don't understand why she didn't like the session. Modesty aside, I was brilliant!

[*The two of them leave the stage and then return, giving the impression that another session has begun*]

DORA: [*Smiling, almost victorious, she announces*]: Dr Freud, today is December 31, 1900, our last session! I'm ending the treatment. New century, new life! I'm grateful for what you've done for me. I know that you made every effort. But I wanted support, someone I can share my anxieties with. Someone who believes in me.

FREUD: My job as an analyst is to reveal your unconscious. Only in this way will you be able to overcome your symptoms. As long as you deny the deep feelings you hold inside yourself, you won't get better.

DORA: Then I'll stay alone in my house, in my room, with my reading. I wanted an ally. A few times you almost were, but then . . . No one understands me. Maybe my brother Otto, with his socialist ideas . . . He belongs to the Austrian Socialist Party. He's been telling me about the falseness of the bourgeois family and the injustices of the capitalist system. [*Getting up from the divan, she feels moved. She extends her hand in a friendly way*] Dr Freud, I give you my sincere thanks and wish you much success in the new year, in the new century! [*She leaves the stage*]

[*Freud remains in silence, motionless. This silence must reverberate on the stage. He returns slowly, and with his shoulders slightly hunched, goes to the desk and writes*]

Scene 8

[*stage left*]

My dear Fliess, she has stopped the treatment. She left like . . . she couldn't care less. We had only eleven sessions. I confess that I was disappointed, sad even. I know that a patient's resistance can explain abandoning treatment. But, in truth, I didn't master the transference. I forgot to be careful to pay attention to the first signs of transference. Transference is more than mere resistance. It seems to me that her father and Mr K's disapproval concealed her own self-disapproval. That accusatory logic hid a profound passion. At certain times, I was willing to believe what she said, but in psychoanalysis, the psychic truth comes before the true story. She felt my neutrality to be a lack of allegiance. The progress of psychoanalysis in this new century will bring answers that I don't yet have. The most interesting thing, for us, in the next century, is perhaps the fact that it contains the date of our death. Fliess, [*as if ending a speech*] I'm going to embark on a sublimation: I'll write about this case and transform a clinical failure into a scientific triumph.

[*The director of the scene or a banner announces: "Fifteen years later"*]

Scene 9

[*Setting: Open space. A sign: "Augarten Park". Moreno wears a long dark-green robe that reaches almost to his ankles. He appears to be watching children playing. Dora goes by, returns a few steps and approaches*]

DORA: Are you Dr Jacob Levy?

MORENO: [*He always speaks in a somewhat discursive, lecturing, slightly maniac tone*] That's me, but you can call me Moreno. And I'm not a doctor yet – I graduate next year.

DORA: I'm Ida Bauer, but you can call me Dora. I've heard that you help people . . .

MORENO: I try, I try. Along with some friends, among them Chaim Kellmer. Do you know Chaim? [*Dora shakes her head*]

MORENO: Great guy, great guy! We founded the encounter religion, the encounter house. I helped prostitutes get organized into a type of union. For some time I've been trying to make these kids [*he points to the park*] unlearn the old children's stories, modify them, and create others. I bring down the cultural conserves – I bring them down! Here the children play little games, like going around the park looking for "new parents". You can't imagine, Chaim chose me as his "new father"! Here I teach disobedience. It is at least as, if not more important than obedience.

DORA: But isn't it dangerous?

MORENO: Nothing ventured, nothing gained, my lady. That is to say, those who aren't daring, fossilize. Those who don't flow with spontaneity, don't create. And soon, young lady, I'll be going to the Mittendorf refugee camp. Now there's a real mess! I'm going to try to organize them in groups according to attractions, repulsions and indifferences. You have no idea how these microsocial networks . . .

DORA: [*Cutting off what she supposes will be a long explanation about sociometry*] What brings me here is that I continue to suffer from the same symptoms. A few years ago I tried doing psychoanalysis with Dr Freud, but I have nothing good to say about it.

MORENO: You really seem to be an intelligent person. Anything that Dr Freud may have done with you, in principal, I am against, totally against! But, how can I help?

[*Background music. We see Dora's silhouette as she recounts her story and Moreno's surprised, slightly exaggerated reactions*]

MORENO: [*In a thoughtful tone*] But you should have followed your feminist and socialist inclinations. You would have found your deeper identity and freed yourself of your symptoms. A social cure! Because this isn't about an individual sickness, but rather a group, family, social one. You aren't the only sick one. It's the relational network that's sick. My God, a sea of transference! Everyone will have to come. We could do an open session right here in the park. Even Dr Freud should come. Everyone involved in this sextet. [*He makes a pun by pronouncing "sex-tet"*] We'll do a "reciprocal theater", a *milieu thérapie*. The real symbol of therapeutic theater is the home. There the theater arises in its most profound sense, because our deepest secrets violently resist being touched upon and exposed. The first house, the place where life begins and ends, the house of birth and death, the house of the most intimate interpersonal relations, becomes the stage and setting. The proscenium is the front door, window and porch. The audience is in the yard and the street. When two people live together and see each other every day, then the real theatrical situation begins. But from this labyrinth of complications with mother and father, wife and son, friend and enemy, built up over a whole lifetime, which winds up changing the person's own world in virtue of insights and misunderstandings, comes, at last, a question: how can they be saved? And all must be saved because all are genuine parts of existence that arise spontaneously. And this is what can be done through the ultimate theater: therapeutic theater. The whole past is exhumed from its grave and responds immediately to the call. It doesn't emerge only to cure itself, for relief and catharsis, but it's also the love of it's own demons that leads the theater to free itself from its shackles. In order to escape from their prisons, people open their deepest, most secretive wounds and bleed externally, in front of our eyes. The whole community is the spectator to therapeutic theater. But this crazy passion, this revelation of life in the dominion of illusion, doesn't work as a revelation of suffering; on the contrary, it confirms the general rule: every true second time is the liberation of the first. The first time makes the second overflow with joy. Every living person denies himself and resolves himself through psychodrama. Life and psychodrama mutually compensate and end in joy. It's theater's final form. And, according to this analysis, a catharsis occurs: not just for the public – a desired secondary effect – and not just in the personal dramas of an imaginary production but, primarily, in the spontaneous actors of the drama who produce the characters, liberating themselves from them at the same time.

DORA: Wow, you speak so beautifully! But does your method really work; can it really cure?

MORENO: My dear, I'm not worried about curing. My concern is with the spontaneous flow among people. You might even continue with your neurosis as long as you creatively transform your way of relating to yourself and to others. There is also the possibility that other people: your father, your mother, or Mr and Mrs K would be able to flex the hardened ties that bind them.

DORA: So, wouldn't it be better for this reunion session to take place at my parent's house?

MORENO: Excellent! Great! You've understood perfectly the meaning of my words! You're a born psychodramatist! At your parent's house, exactly! Psychodrama *in situ*. As I've said, in its *locus*. Dora, I feel we have affinity. Actually, it's a shame you're already married, because I've been looking for a muse [*he makes a romantic, in-love face*] to inspire my life, my work. But this is another story, for another time. So, it's all set: at your parent's house. I hope they'll all be there!

[*The stage darkens. A spotlight focuses on the director of the spontaneous-psychodrama theater. He explains that "tonight (or this afternoon) is improvised". The regular actors, as well as the soon-to-be spontaneous actors from the audience, will perform Act II. Now the creation belongs to everyone. Everyone becomes the author and actors. The stage is illuminated again. We see empty chairs, which will be filled by the characters, arranged in a semicircle. The director warms up the audience and starts filling the chairs. After this intermediary scene, others may follow*]

Act II

Spontaneous theater psychodrama

Group creation

The end

Sources

Freud, S. (1968). *Análisis fragmentario de una histeria*. Obras completas, vol. II. Madrid: Biblioteca Nueva. (English edition: *Fragment of an analysis of a case of hysteria*. Complete psychological works of Sigmund Freud, vol. VII, pp. 51–52. London: Hogarth Press, 1905.)

Gay, P. (1989). *Freud, uma vida para o nosso tempo*. São Paulo: Companhia das Letras. (Original edition: *Freud: a life for our time*. New York/London: Norton, 1988.)

Masson, J. M. (ed.) (1986). *Correspondência Sigmund Freud–Wilhem Fliess*. Rio de Janeiro: Imago. (Original edition: *The complete letters of Sigmund Freud to Wilhelm Fliess, 1877–1904*. London: Belknap Press of Harvard University Press, 1985.)

Moreno, J. L. (1977). *Psychodrama – First Volume* (5th edn). New York: Beacon House, Inc.

Rodrigué, E. (1995). *Sigmund Freud. O século da psicanálise: 1895–1995 (Sigmund Freud. The century of psychoanalysis: 1895–1995)*. São Paulo: Escuta.

Chapter 9

Public psychodrama

*José Fonseca, Maria Amalia Faller Vitele
and Mery Candido de Oliveira*

Open sessions

The first time I watched a public psychodrama was in 1967, during the
Latin-American Group Psychotherapy Congress in São Paulo, Brazil. It
took place in the Catholic University Theater (TUCA) and was directed by
Rojas-Bermudez. There were great repercussions throughout the local
psychiatric community. I was surprised by the way the people denuded
themselves psychologically and by the spontaneous way in which the
audience interacted with the protagonists. I have since, as a psychodramatist, watched and directed innumerable public psychodramas. But
nothing has ever impressed me as much as the open sessions held at the
Moreno Institute in Beacon in 1979. What most enchanted me were the
participants who went in search of psychotherapeutic help. Unlike my
previous experiences, in which the groups were comprised primarily of
professionals in the fields of psychology, in Beacon the audience was made
up preponderantly of lay people, uninterested in learning psychodrama
techniques. This American experience led to the initiation, in 1984, of open
psychotherapy sessions at the Daimon-Center for Relationship Studies[1]
(the entity that I coordinate in São Paulo), which still continue today.

   The fact that this chapter is included in "New Approaches to Psychodrama Technique" reveals that the oldest form of psychodrama (remember
Moreno in Vienna on April 1, 1921) can always be renewed just as Moreno
said about spontaneity, "it is an appropriate response to a new situation or
a new response to an old situation".

---

1 Daimon-Center for Relationship Studies is a non-profit organization whose purpose is to
  foster personal development, in addition to the training of professionals, in the areas of
  psychology and psychiatry. Yet another objective is community assistance, including the
  organization of psychotherapeutic or psychoprophylactic activities aimed at the public.

Reflecting the experience

> I come to the open sessions in search of magic. Only here do I have the
> chance to meet people in a way that doesn't happen outside. They are
> strangers and yet so close.
>
> An open-session participant

Maria Amalia Faller Vitale
Mery Candido de Oliveira

This text stems from reflections on the open psychotherapy sessions, which
have taken place at the Daimon-Center since 1984. During this time, as
members of the coordinating team, we have gathered statements from the
protagonists and audience participants, consulted the session registers and
held evaluation meetings with the therapists involved in the work.

While re-examining and organizing the data, the questions and obstacles
that arose led us to attempt to align this practical experience to some initial
theoretical points. Our hope, thus, is to outline this dimension of psychodramatic work that, though central to psychodrama, has been little explored.

Returning to the origins

First, we will briefly review Moreno's work with theater, which came into
his life early on. While still young, he created the "Theater of Spontaneity"
in Vienna. His objective, in addition to denouncing the political and social
situation in post-First World War Vienna, was to propose improvisational
theater, inspired by the model developed by the *commedia dell'arte* and the
Comédie-Française in the sixteenth and seventeenth centuries. The primary
characteristics of the two theater groups were improvised plays, without
written scripts; fixed actors performing the same roles, sometimes for their
entire lifetime; and themes based on the hunger–love–money triangle. Most
times, the content, despite a burlesque presentation, contained social criticism adapted to the specific characteristics of the region where the play was
being presented.

Moreno's *theater of spontaneity* incorporated both social significance and
the elimination of the playwright and written text from Italian and French
comedies. Moreno (1976, p. 49) intended for the actors and audience to be
one, working in "an open space, the space of life, life itself".

Later, through the "Barbara Case", Moreno discovered the therapeutic
possibilities of role-play. *Spontaneous theater* led to *therapeutic theater*.

We return to Moreno's thoughts on the meaning of therapeutic theater:

> The theatre for spontaneity was the unchaining of illusion. But this
> illusion acted out by the people who have lived through it in reality, is

the unchaining of life – "das Ding ausser sich". The theatre of the last things is not the eternal recurrence of the same, out of eternal necessity (Nietzsche), but the opposite of it. *It is the self produced and self created recurrence of itself.*

(Moreno, 1973, p. 92)

Open sessions incorporate the meaning of therapeutic theater, correlating theater and life. They reveal to the audience, through quotidian scenes, the intimacy of interpersonal relations. The *second-time* experience contains the possibility of a therapeutic dimension. On the other hand, since it is a type of work whose compromise (among director, protagonist and audience) lasts for one session only and which is over with the end of the session, this therapeutic dimension occurs through a therapeutic act.

Open sessions are, therefore, both intimately connected to the origins of psychodrama itself and, at the same time, would appear to be an innovative proposal, if the current development of psychodramatic work is taken as a reference.

Characterizing the work

In 1984 open psychotherapy sessions were initiated at the Daimon-Center. José Fonseca, coordinator of this entity, comments:

> Despite knowing through of the activities Moreno developed at the therapeutic theater in New York City and Beacon, only in 1979 was I able to watch the presentations in Beacon personally. The "open sessions" were held on Saturday nights. The audience consisted of injured Vietnam veterans, university students, neighborhood residents and participants of the psychodrama training group at the Moreno Institute. I was fascinated by the experience. I imagined that, if there were any way, I would try to do it in Brazil.
>
> (interview in 1988)

On May 10, 1984, José Fonseca directed the first open session at the Daimon-Center. The initial objectives of the open sessions were to offer an alternative to therapeutic work; to reach a population group with less access to private therapy; and to foster the learning of different therapeutic directing techniques.

The sessions, about two hours long, were moved to Thursday nights at the Daimon Therapeutic Theater. They were open to the public for a modest fee; participants were not required to sign up in advance. The therapists invited by the coordinating team worked primarily with action methods.

Initially, putting together the director's schedule for the sessions was no easy task; many therapists refused, others asked for some time to get used to the idea. Among the therapists who made the proposal viable during the first year, we highlight a few: José Fonseca (psychodrama), Luis Altenfelder (psychodrama), Antonio Gonçalves (psychodrama), Alfredo Naffah (psychodrama), A. C. Godoy (bioenergetics), J. A. Gaiarsa (neo-reichian therapy), Luiz Cuschnir (psychodrama), Saulo Berber (gestalt therapy), Maria Melo (bioenergetics), Oswaldo de Souza Junior (psycho-drama), Marcelo Campedelli (psychodrama), Regina Favre (neo-reichian therapy) and Leonardo Satne (psychoanalytic psychodrama).

The coordinating team tried announcing the sessions at a few of the social nuclei and mental health centers in the neighborhoods near Daimon, though these announcements appeared to reach few. In fact, resources previously utilized by Daimon (flyers, programs, posters) proved the most effective advertising. Later on, the members of the audience themselves let others know of the sessions.

Again, the proposal was to offer an alternative therapy to those uncon-nected to psychodrama or other therapies, rather than to meet the teaching needs of psychodrama students.

The public

Reports made from 1986 to 1988 allow an initial profile of the people who attended the open sessions to be configured.

Number of people who participated in the activity

- *1986*: From March to November (eight months) 979 people attended, 369 for the first time.
- *1987*: From March to November (eight months) 953 people attended, 381 for the first time.
- *1988*: From March to June (four months) 344 people attended, 136 for the first time.

Geographic reach

From a sample of 122 people taken during June 1988 it was observed that the public frequenting the sessions resided primarily in middle-class neigh-borhoods. Perhaps the most relevant information obtained, however, is that the open sessions reached a broad public, which included people coming for the first time.

The observations of the coordinating team, together with the studies conducted, also indicate that the audience is subdivided into three categ-ories: those participating for the first time; those who participate occasionally; and those who comprise a subgroup of people who participate weekly, forming a parallel therapeutic "process", once a group or subgroup dynamic has been established. These subgroups are stable and last about a year on average. From 1984 to 1988 three different formations took place. The groups begin in a similar way: starting at a particular session, generally one of protagonization, an individual begins to frequent the sessions weekly, grouping himself with others who have already participated. Within a year, more or less, this subgroup breaks up and another begins to form from the remaining members. There are several people who have participated in the open sessions for many years, moving through various subgroups.

This seems to demonstrate that the open sessions, being a regular activity, tend to foster the formation of nuclei of habitual participants, thus forming some particular processual characteristics. From this a few questions arise: to what extent does this subgroup direct the group work since the therapists, who rotate every week (they are invited to direct one session), are unaware of its formation? Do these subgroups perform a therapeutic process? If so, what are the characteristics of this process?

Another aspect worthy of comment is that there are a significant number of professionals in the area of psychology who frequent the sessions. Even though the initial objective of the open sessions was not to provide work models, this happened anyway.

The therapists

The team of professionals who direct the open sessions at the Daimon-Center is made up of therapists from the institution itself as well as outside "guests". The line of work, in general, is linked to action methods and group work (psychodrama, bioenergetics, gestalt, transactional analysis).

The greatest challenge for an open-session therapist seems to be working with the unknown. The therapist has no previous history with the protagonist or the group. He/she works with the protagonist suggested by the group. It is a meeting of two strangers with a common goal, established within the *telic–transferential* sphere. This yields the following questions: what are the chances of establishing a *telic* or *transferential* relationship, since the director doesn't choose the protagonist? And what are the *telic*, *transferential* and *counter-transferential* aspects involved like?

Some psychodramatists have their first, or at least some significant, psychodramatic experiences with open sessions. Others, on the other hand, have never had the experience. This leads to some considerations since many psychodramatists go through their professional training without this (therapeutic theater) experience – such an essential part of psychodrama.

Other issues to be considered are the following:

- The type of psychodramatic training.
- The psychodramatic model demanded by the job market.
- The theoretical model which emphasizes processual psychodramatic psychotherapy.
- The privacy of the therapist's office, where his/her working methods are sheltered (they are not exposed to the public).

The protagonist

The protagonist that emerges in an open group has been warming-up since the moment he decided to go to the open session. "I denominate this prior process 'warm-up'. Fantasies appear with respect to what may happen during the session or with the expressed desire to be the protagonist or with reactive attitudes" (Bustos, 1974, p. 39).

We have observed, and the statements of some therapists corroborate, that long warm-ups retard the emergence of the protagonist. This occurs, perhaps, because the group energy is directed to the warm-up and to the group work, taking the focus away from the problematic individual.

Commonly, the protagonist communicates that he/she has never done therapy or psychodramatic work. Some protagonists emerge not only as a sociometric expression of the public, but also because they would like to be treated by a determined therapist. In this case, perhaps the first protagonist is the director him/herself. A comment frequently made in the area of psychodrama is that this public work favors the emergence of protagonists with hysterical personality traits. The question is whether this makes the work more difficult or requires another type of technical management. Some protagonists seem to need a large audience (which mobilizes energy and emotion) as a container for their dramas. The protagonist needs the complement of the audience. The protagonist leaves the audience in order to be seen and heard by it. Soeiro (1990), referring to this, speaks of *audience instinct*. The theme most frequently presented by the public pro-tagonist is *relationship–separation* (marital separation, death, family conflicts). Some of these scenes lead to the sub-theme of *sexuality*.

It is interesting to observe that the protagonists who work with mourning or childhood sexual experiences seem to need the presence of the audience, which acts as a resonance box, even more than others. Does public work offer more elements for the elaboration of the mourning ritual? It seems as if the mourning ritual in itself, when not experienced in life, is better elaborated when relived together with the therapeutic theater audience; that is, when it takes place within the collective realm.

Another point to be mentioned refers to the psychosocial dynamic relative to the public exposition of childhood sexual experiences to the expression of intimacy. Are these experiences more efficiently atoned for if we approach them in terms of the presence of guilt (which is also questionable)? Or do the protagonists seek the public's allegiance against sexual aggressions of the past? Or does unveiling such *guarded* scenes mean breaking from the dominance and tyranny of privacy?

The public and the private

The public–private relationship is at the heart of therapeutic theater. Naffah observes:

> Each discourse is initially presented as absolutely personal and private, reigning over the collective being which sustains it. But absolute privacy means absolute solitude, emptiness, death . . . The protagonist is thus the spokesperson of the Drama, his action and speech condensing the collective being which sustains the action and discourse of each one and of all.
>
> (Naffah, 1982, p. 57)

At open sessions, the interrelationship of the individual with the social is constructed as the protagonist's sociometric choices are made during the unfolding of the scenes. It is, however, during the *sharing* stage that the public, in manifesting the private, salvages the collective and breaks from the isolation of privacy. At this moment, the protagonist reveals not only his/her intimacy but also that which is contained in the group, in the collective.

It is from these co-existing and contradictory dimensions that the feeling of the open sessions arises: "I like to come; I always wind up realizing that problems are similar and that we are not so original. I end up treating myself too" (statement of a participant).

Through sharing, sadness and happiness, relationships and separation, and life and death reconfigure the dominance of the meaning of the individual. The loneliness of privacy is broken. The open session comes to an end.

What follows is a condensed report of an open session, conducted by the author, with sixty-eight participants.

Warm-up

The theater is full so the director asks the participants to try to find a comfortable position in their seats, reduce the flow of their thoughts and movements, pay attention to their bodies, prioritizing the prevailing sensations, and beginning from there, allow visual images to manifest themselves.

After a few minutes, he asks the people who would like to work with their internally visualized image or scene to approach him. Each person briefly presents his scene and then the sociometric choice of a protagonist is made. In this case, the protagonist is a middle-aged woman with a shy appearance, soberly dressed. She reports that she came to the open session with the idea of being directed by José Fonseca, looking to "treat" her unhappiness. The idea arose when she saw another person working with a similar situation in an *open session* directed by him. The protagonist had undergone processual psychotherapy but hadn't overcome her symptoms.

Dramatization (action)

The scene visualized in the warm-up is a door in front of a small country home, which the protagonist is unable to open. The feeling present is sadness.

Scene I

The protagonist assembles the family's country home and places herself at the door. In soliloquy, she speaks of the house as a project of the couple and the family, of her husband's hard work and dreams, of the time it took to build the house; she also speaks of the overwhelming sadness she feels when she goes there, to the point where she is unable to remain in the house. She remembers her husband dying in a car accident, with the country home yet to be opened. At the time of her husband's death, she was unable to see him since the coffin had been sealed shut; she had also not been permitted to look at the photos of the accident taken by the police.

Scene II

The director asks if she would like to "go" to the accident. She does. She re-enacts the accident, reconstructing her husband's route (role reversal) on the road, up to the moment of the crash. The scene unfolds with the audience reproducing the sound of the motors and the noise of the cars hitting until the husband finds himself near death. Through the performance of role reversal, the husband says how much he loves her and the family and the pain he feels in being unable to fulfill their dreams. She is included in the scene (then in the role of herself) in order to say goodbye to her husband. She reports her anger at being abandoned, the sadness she feels, the pain of being alone and her love for him. She participated in the scene until his death. The director asks if the husband can go away to the "other side" and be released from the "living-dead". She agrees. She returns to the first scene, contemplating the country home and the future from a new perspective.

The group shares common situations and feelings with the protagonist. The sharing is the last step of the open session.

Open sessions, in this case, seem to be a space in which pain can be shared and suffering socialized. People break away from their quotidian lives, offering a new context for the protagonist to relive his/her deaths and work through another level of mourning. It is possible, in this way, to change the "quality of the pain", as was affirmed by a participant of these sessions.

References

Bustos, D. M. (1974). *El psicodrama (Psychodrama)*. Buenos Aires: Plus Ultra.

Moreno, J. L. (1973). *The theater of spontaneity*. New York: Beacon House, Inc.

Moreno, J. L. (1976). *Psicodrama*. São Paulo: Cultrix. (Original edition: *Psychodrama – First Volume*. New York: Beacon House, Inc., 1946).

Naffah Neto, A. (1982). *As psicoterapias hoje. Algumas abordagens (Psychotherapies today. Some approaches)*. São Paulo: Summus.

Soeiro, A. C. (1990). *O instinto de platéia (The audience instinct)*. Porto: Afrontamento.

Part 3

Psychodrama and sexuality

Chapter 10

Sexuality as a relational instrument*

Sex is a great mystery.

Henry Miller, *The World of Sex*

Invited to speak about psychosexual development to sex therapists, I became aware of the exercises recommended to improve sexual dysfunction. It then occurred to me to reflect upon the relationship of *I* with itself (*I–I*) and of *I* with *you*, with the *other* (*I–you*) in terms of sexual development. Which phases of psychosexual evolution would influence (and how) sexual function and dysfunction? Moreno doesn't approach sexuality in a specific way. He offers a broad theory on existential character and an objective technique, psychodrama, for the study of sexuality. In one of his few references on sexuality he comments, "The bodily attachment of infant to mother is a forerunner of the later behavior in the sexual role" (Moreno, 1977, p. v). In "The Warming Up Process in the Sexual Act" (Moreno, 1977, p. 206), he proposes the psychodramatic method in approaching sexual dysfunctions.[1]

Psychodrama, psychoanalysis and sexuality

I start from the point of view that the human relationship, as a whole, precedes sexuality. Man is motivated by the *relational instinct*. Sexuality is one of his relational instruments, and sexual disorders would thus be responsible for one part of relational disorders. Sexual disorder belongs,

* My thanks to Moacir Costa who, in inviting me innumerable times to speak about sexuality and psychodrama, incited me to write on the subject, and to Fátima Fontes for her excellent suggestions and stimulation on the final draft.
1 Ronaldo Pamplona da Costa in verbal communication at SGM (Study Group on Moreno) – Daimon, highlights the pioneering nature of this approach, at least twenty years before the sex therapy techniques of Masters and Johnson.

therefore, to a greater relational difficulty that is manifested, given certain circumstances, sexually. Opposing Freud's classic collocation of sexuality, even at the beginning of a new century with imminent new ideas, is no easy task.

I accept Freudian psychodynamics in essence, when relieved of exaggeration in relation to sexuality and the Oedipus complex. In my clinical hypotheses, I dispense with the ego, id and superego. I prefer to think in terms of a *global I*, composed of innumerable *partial I(s)*, including *censoring I(s)*, which express themselves through both latent and emergent roles.[2] The constellation (cluster) of *partial I(s)* which constitutes the *global sexual I* is expressed through sexual roles, which contain psychosomatic, psychological and social components in their structure. In my understanding of the unconscious, I have trouble accepting the Freudian assertion that words come before images, even taking into account that this concept was formulated before the advent of movies and television. My conception of *energy* is more like Moreno's spontaneity-creativity than Freud's libido. The notion of libido is tied to the concepts of classical physics and thermodynamics, understood as a storable category of energy. Spontaneity, on the other hand, is conceived as something both *storable* and *nonstorable*, more in accordance with a systemic vision and the principles of quantum physics; that is, the more spontaneity is liberated, the more it is created. Finally, I understand the Freudian "life and death instincts" to have three positions, not two. Freud allows that, besides a destructive tendency, there is the human being's creative impulse of transcendence. But I imagine that it would be more didactic to consider a *constructive instinct*, a *destructive instinct*, and a *transcendental instinct*, that seeks *nothing*, peace, and that represents a longing for the essence, the period before and after (death) the personality. This corresponds to the states of consciousness reached through meditation, or through experiences in the *no-thought* sphere of internal emptiness. The transcendental instinct is responsible for man's mysticism and his/her search for the sacred. Even an atheist can be mystical, because curiosity and respect for a greater universal dimension ("mystery" and "mystical" have the same root) are part of his/her essence. I believe that this component should be distinguished from the death instinct due to the qualitative differences that it presents.

I believe that one of Freud's most important psychological characteristics was his seriousness. As I made reference to in another section, our personality traits have both a positive and a negative side. Seriousness, in its positive aspect, gave Freud scientific consistency and professional credibility. However, the exaggeration of this trait, aggravated by a long illness, was revealed by his skepticism and bitterness, which probably made his

2 Perazzo (1986) discusses the "sexual" role and its development up to the encounter.

work more somber than it would have been otherwise. Though Freud once stated in an interview that he wasn't pessimistic, one would hardly say that his work emanated cheer. I believe that his vision of sexuality, as a consequence, failed to receive a more relaxed treatment, and that the connection of sexuality to aesthetics and beauty was less emphasized than it could have been.

The integration between love and sexuality must also be acknowledged. Love is part of a broader process that involves the opposite of love: hate – at the other pole of the established relationship. The *love/hate* process concerns the psychological sphere of the loving relationship. Sexuality concerns its biological sphere. This (merely didactic) division signifies that in a sexual relationship, from a psychological point of view, the *love/hate* process is always involved. Some argue that there can be sex without love. However, conceptually, the *love/hate* process entails all relationships in which sexuality is present.

Loving relationship can also be understood from a relational–sociometric position in which there are both congruent and incongruent reciprocal choices in positive, negative and neutral terms. These choices generate different reactions from the people involved: pleasure, happiness, sadness, anger, indifference, etc. Thus, so-called "sex without love", or with "unlove", or with hatred, always has the *love/hate* process implicit. I employ the word *love*, then, in a broad sense and the word *sex* in a specific one.

The simple observation that sexual relations are the most intimate physical contact between two people leads to an understanding of its symbolic potential. This proximity causes occasional conflicts, which may be present in one partner, to emerge in the other or in the relationship between the two. From this perspective, a sexual relationship can be frustrating if one of the elements presents difficulties, if both do, or even if neither did before, if the relationship is harmed by psychological factors inherent to the momentary circumstances.

If we take the physical parameter as a symbol of the psychological, when two people unclothe, show themselves physically with no disguises or artifices, sense each other's scent, mix saliva and mucus, penetrate each other, there is a strong *energetic* exchange.

Imagine two people face to face, a few feet from each other. They are nude and looking at each other. They slowly approach. When they are near, they touch and embrace, beginning to lay the foundation. Now go back to the first image: the two approaching each other. Imagine that one begins to feel fear or distrust. His or her body shrinks and avoids the other who, in turn, also falters. As they get closer, one or both retreat, surprised. By studying the symbolism of the movement of their bodies we can know, in some way, what these people are like. For example, in a heterosexual relationship, a man reveals himself not only within the context of the relationship with that specific woman but also in the context of relationships with women in general, and, in a greater context, with the world. We have, then, three concentric circles: the sexual relationship with a specific person of the opposite sex, the sexual relationship with people of the opposite sex, and the generic relationship with all other human beings.

Sexuality as a relational instrument

Adult personality traits are sculpted by experiences from the phases of neuropsychological development. In this period, the psychological configurations that represent the person and give him/her identity (*trademark*) are formed. The concept of sexual development in phases follows from the notion that layers of psychological events, experienced and internalized, are superimposed over the energetic essence with which one is born. One could imagine these phases of psychosocial influence superimposing themselves concentrically, similar to the way in which a tree grows – the tree trunk is the personality or *I* and the branches are the social roles of adult life. The roles (branches) come from exactly the same structure as the personality (trunk).

The roles are the arms of the personality and serve in relationships with counter-roles (roles, arms or branches of other people). In studying one of a person's social roles, one studies, in a way, his/her personality too, as both have the same structures. A complete study requires the observation of expressed and latent roles and of the clusters (Moreno, 1977) of roles. In this way, one knows what the "tree" is like in the present and infers the history of its development.

The study of sexual roles follows the same procedure. Sexual roles, like all others, are comprised of psychosomatic roles, fantasy or imaginary roles (psychological or psychodramatic roles for Moreno) and social roles. Psychosomatic roles represent the biological base, fantasy roles signify the psychological structure, and social roles bring social and cultural impregnation to sexuality.

For the presentation of the psychological development phases, which run from birth until adulthood, I utilize the scheme revealed in Chapter 1 of this book. I make use of Moreno's (1961) concept of the *matrix of identity* as a base for these psychosocial dynamic contributions. The following phases of the matrix of identity are utilized in the study of sexuality: indifferentiation, symbiosis, recognition of I, recognition of you, corridor relationship, pre-inversion of roles or performance of the role of the other, triangulation, circularization, role reversal and the encounter. Some have been used as a base while others have been left out in this description of new phases. The phases are dynamic, with alternations and successions, and don't necessarily follow a chronological order. As Wechsler (1997) underlines, this approach is not linear but rather "spiral", analogous to the study of knowledge construction. In 1935, Melanie Klein (1996) coined the term "phase" to substitute the word "position". I propose adopting this change to make clear that these configurations belong not only to childhood but also make up part of the adult psyche. My purpose is to establish correlations between the phases of psychosexual development and the way one is in adult loving (sexual) relationships.

Sexual indifferentiation

From the time a child is born up to a certain period of life, he/she is unaware of his/her sexual identity. He/she doesn't know if he/she is male or female. He/she lives an existential mixture or, one could say, a unilateral symbiosis with his/her mother.

Relationship/separation

In this phase, the child begins the *learning of relationship/separation* (bonding). This learning makes up the structural foundation of the roles involved in loving relationships. In other words, the child learns the pairs of opposites essential for life: relationship/separation, love/rejection, being rejected/rejecting, love/hate and all the variations, arrangements and ways of accommodating these psychological structures. With this list of internalized answers, he/she will respond to adult sexual choices (to choose and be chosen).

When the child is still under six months of age, he/she demonstrates an unspecified attraction to humans. It doesn't matter if these people are known or not; he/she doesn't possess the neuropsychological discrimination necessary for such selection. Direct observations of a baby demonstrate his/her natural attraction for human sounds and shapes. Little by little, the child begins to discriminate between *known* and *unknown* people (tele); within a determined period, the child "elects" (bonds with) preferred people who provide tranquility, security and pleasure. With these "elected" people, the child learns the pleasure of relationship and the pain of separation. At the first sign of separation, he/she reacts with an observable list of emotional reactions: anxiety, anger and sadness. He/she then returns to his/her normal state, elaborates the loss and begins to learn about the separation process, thus beginning the formation of behaviors to avoid the pain of separation: *defense mechanisms* (*shock-absorbers*) of *separation–loss*.

Sexual attraction is comparable to an internal light that is turned on, regardless of place or circumstances. It exists at the edge of rational discernment or desire; it is instinctive, despite being permeated by cultural values. Sexual attraction, diffuse in puberty, becomes defined by preferred figures (boyfriend, girlfriend, husband–wife, lover–lover) according to the sociometry of sex.

In order for the choice to be concretized, there must be a positive counterpart from *the other* (sociometry in two). In this situation, the anxiety–fear–desperation of separation (rejection) arises and, unless counter-chosen, *anger–hatred* and *sadness–depression* also appear. Defense mechanisms, absorbers of psychological pain, then come into play. These experiences, just like in the childhood *matrix of identity*, define the day-to-day experiences of sexual attractions and loving relationships.

The ideal sexual I

In going through the phases of the *matrix of identity*, the existential sexual and relational identity of the individual is processed. As mentioned in Chapter 4, at a certain phase of the matrix of identity, the record that the baby is beautiful, admired and loved preponderates. In the words of Kohut (1984), the baby registers "the shine in his mother's eyes." This energetic impregnation develops and imprints a sensation of grandiosity and exhibitionism in the baby.[3] On the other hand, when this fails to occur, the baby feels "cut off" from these inebriating sensations and is immersed in the pain provoked by this "wound". The balance–imbalance of this duality (relation/separation, love/rejection, pleasure/pain) represents the point on the scale that divides the healthy (self-esteem and tolerance toward frustration) from the pathological (identity disorders). In this way, the rudiments of an *ideal I* (always loved and admired), in contrast to the *I*, begin to arise – the *be–appear* dyad is initiated. The self-image is either firmed or obscured depending on the inputs received from *the other*, which, in turn, comes to be discriminated or confused with an *ideal you*, a *frustrating you* or simply *you*.

These first childhood experiences are transformed and relived in loving relationships. The object of our love is toasted with the shine in our eyes. And we receive *the shine in our partner's eyes*, which makes us feel we are the most beautiful, most seductive, etc. The absence of this shine leaves us sad or angry. (Deep inside, everyone wants to be considered the best lover.) The individual creates a self-concept of how good a lover he/she is. This tension can motivate the search for perfection or lead to a compulsive search for an intangible sexual performance.

An example of this dynamic can be seen in a patient who relates his fear of remarrying. His justification is that his previous wives made his life hell. All of them were madly in love, jealous and possessive. He wasn't in love with any of them, instead being in love with their passion (for him). He

---

3 Williams observes that this phase of development would fit in with Moreno's expression: *normal megalomania*. But he adds, "as the years pass, we all see ourselves forced to become more humble" (1994, p. 259).

needed the mad but passionate shine in these women's eyes. At these times he felt in heaven, though he paid the price of matrimonial hell.

Corridor relationships

A child, in the *corridor relationship* phase, forms exclusive and possessive relationships. He/she already has an identity and distinguishes the other, but feels that the other exists only for him/her. There are memories of the child's recent past in which he/she felt "as one" (symbiosis) with his/her mother. He/she feels unique and central in the relationship. In this phase, the child only has eyes for the mother and wants the mother's eyes only for him/her.

The imprints from this phase reappear, in a way, in loving relationships. They are characterized by the desire for exclusivity and, in a distorted way, by the possession of and obsession for the other (*you*). Crimes of passion demonstrate the compulsive aspects of *corridor relationships*. The adult fantasy of possessing a companion completely and definitively originates from these primary experiences. One leaves the relationship with his/her mother (or matrix of identity), grows up, and finds another similar or equal relationship, forever. Or one desires a partner who compensates for what wasn't experienced before, what was missing. The search for the partner–mother (matrix), regardless of one's sex, connotes, in principle, the failure of something that can no longer be obtained.

Loving passion presents a psychological structure based on *corridor relationships*. Passion is a state of exaltation, an "inebriation" of love, where the drug is the other. From a healthy point of view, this means the organismic celebration of two beings who come together. The presence of two sets of internal biochemical reactions provokes alterations in the state of consciousness ("inebriation"). This psychochemical (alchemic?) short-circuit has a limited duration. The next phase is either love or disillusion (the love "hang over"). There is healthy and pathological passion. I denote the former *telic* passion and the latter *transferential* passion – characterized by the projection of unresolved archaic longings onto the new companion. *Transferential passion* confers a magical, savior value to the *other*, with the subsequent frustration when the proof of quotidian reality takes over. *Transferential passion* signifies the persistence of regressive bonds, not their transformation. *Telic passion* is *reversive*; as will be seen in Chapter 12, "Sexual Sociometry and Forms of Sexuality", it transcends the past and presents itself as an enriching experience in the present.

The climax of *telic passion* is the exaltation of life. The peak of *transferential passion* is the exaltation of death. These concepts are eloquently depicted in the film *Empire of the Senses*, by the Japanese director N. Oshima, which portrays the consumption of two lovers until death.

Recognition of the sexual I

This phase refers to the period in which the child becomes aware of his/her own body and genitals. He/she realizes the difference between the two sexes and thus, his/her own sexual identity: *I am a boy*; *I am of the masculine sex* or *I am a girl*; *I am of the feminine sex*. The *recognition of the sexual I* phase could also be called the *sexual mirror* phase. From this point on, *gender identity* is formed, understood here as a social construction.

Before *recognition of the sexual I*, the child has already become aware that he/she exists as an individual (existential recognition), separate from the mother or the matrix of identity: *I exist, I am a person distinct from others*. In the practical study of him/herself, the child sees, manipulates, registers bodily sensations, compares him/herself with other children and adults – in short, defines a consciousness of sex and sexuality. The homosexual games of this period denote the self-centered state of sexual knowledge. In this way, the *recognition of the sexual I* can be understood as a natural homosexual phase of development. Masturbation, which is an instrument of sexual self-knowledge, can also be understood as a "homosexual" relationship, to the extent that it is a sex act of *I* with *I* (of the same sex), regardless of the fact that there may be a fantasy of a *you* of the other sex.

The physio-psycho-social aspects involved in the *sexual I* are manifested in three sub-phases or crises. The first corresponds to the childhood period. The second, after a latent period, is manifested in puberty–adolescence, when the body and genitals assume their adult form. The third period occurs in old age, when a new and definitive transformation of sexuality comes out.

Recognition of the sexual you

The *recognition of the sexual you* phase occurs concomitantly to the *recognition of the sexual I* phase. The distinction between the two is merely didactic. Self-knowledge possesses implicit comparative criteria, where similarities and differences with other people are looked for. *How I am* is related to *how others are* – others of both the same and opposite sex. There is a *mirror of oneself* and *a mirror of the other*. The child discovers the definitive differences between masculine and feminine identities, including him/herself in one of them. In childhood this phase is manifested through playing games such as doctor, house, husband–wife, etc., while during adolescence it is manifested by sexual interest, now defined. Childhood games are substituted for the erotic games of adolescence.

The *sexual you* represents the first internalization of the opposite sex. In the case of a boy, for example, the female pattern comes from interacting with the women who belong to his matrix of identity (mother, grandmother, aunts, sisters, etc.). The internalized configuration of the opposite sex in the matrix of identity is an important reference in the choice of future sexual companions. At the extremes, there is the compulsive search for the same childhood patterns or the opposite of them. That is, sexual partners are chosen according to conscious–unconscious criteria, which inevitably go through the matrix of identity.

Pre-inversion of roles or performing the other's role

This phase serves in the continuation of the recognition of *I* and of the *sexual you*. It covers the area of fantasy as training for future sexual acts (prepar-action). I distinguish *imagination-fantasy* from *action-fantasy*. The first entails all the sexual situations imagined to be exciting and pleasurable. The adolescent male fantasizes having sex with a famous actress, the next-door neighbor, with his sister's friend. The girl has sex, in the same way, with the male idol or with her teacher. The *imagination-fantasy* takes place in the interior space. When an adolescent fantasizes a scene, he/she acts out his/her role with some level of expectation or idealization of him/herself and also plays the role of the partner in the imaginary scene. Playing "doctor" or "house" is an *action-fantasy* situation; that is, a spontaneous dramatization with involvement and corporal participation of the other person. Playing *the role of the other* represents internal–external training (role-playing) of both one's own and the complementary sexual role.

Sexual triangulation

Escaping from the maternal symbiotic mixture represents a second birth, a psychological birth. Whereas during conception there is egalitarian participation between father and mother, during gestation, birth and breast-feeding, mother and child interact within an atmosphere of profound inclusiveness. But, at a certain point, for the psychological survival of both, separation is necessary. The *third* (father) figure then appears in order to promote the severing of the psychological umbilical cord and transform the dyad into a trio. In harmonious triangulation development there is a confluence of three forces: the father seeks the child, the child seeks the father, and the mother facilitates their approximation. This psychological rescue forms the basis of sexual identity. A boy receives the energetic impregnation of masculinity. A girl diffuses herself from the maternal mixture and learns to be another woman. This theme will be further explored in the next chapter: "Sexual Identity".

The triangulation phase fosters the basis for comparison–competition. When a child compares himself with another person of the same sex, not only is comparison implicit but competition is also possible, even without victory as a defined objective. Later, the object under dispute becomes clearer. The resolution of this communicational complex occurs with the advent of guilt, through hating the person who is loved, and the birth and internalization of the *censoring I(s)*. Triangulation signifies, therefore, the rupture of the symbiotic egg between the child (the *first*) and the mother (the *second*) by the appearance of the *third*, the father.

The comparative–competitive aspect of triangulation presents a social dimension: jealousy.[4] The physical–sexual characters in the adolescent are compared to cultural standards, which offer stereotypes of beauty and power that serve as a model to be matched. The elements concerning the psychodynamics of the *ideal sexual I*, which have already been commented on, are connected to this topic. This comparison–competition generates anxiety–fear–insecurity. *I need to be better than him so that you will prefer me.* When the (male) *I* is in bed with his *you*, he always feels the *he* prowling around. This situation suggests that there are three tasks: obtain pleasure, offer pleasure, and beat the sexual competitor. The triangulation phase in adolescence is illustrated by the boastful statements of boys. It is as if they were saying: *Look, I'm better than you!* And to themselves: *But I'm still not what I'd like to be.* This dynamic is concreted in the *ménage à trois*. If the partner is the same – that is, also bringing the *third* – there are then four in bed whose concretization is the *swing*.

Sexual circularization

Circularization is most clearly illustrated by small groups chatting and telling secrets about sex. The group gives strength. During childhood, in one way, and in adolescence, in another, conversations about sex receive the complicity of the group. In adulthood, telling sex jokes and gossiping about others' sex lives have the same connotation (circularized sex). Group sex, where all participate and all observe, is also related to this dynamic.

Sexual role reversal

Sexual role reversal signifies the zenith of the sexual development process. It occurs when the man knows the woman and she knows him. It represents the capacity to put oneself at the two poles: the masculine and the feminine, the active and the passive, giving and receiving. It brings with it the possibility of learning the sensitivity of the other sex. It is knowing how to caress with the hand and capture the feeling in the other's body.

4 Consult *Jealousy, the fear of loss* (Ferreira-Santos, 1996).

Sexual encounter[5]

The encounter originates from role reversal. It is a phenomenon of the *telic* apex. The *sexual encounter* precipitates an altered state of consciousness. It is activated by the transcendence of greater sexual excitement. It can occur as much as a consequence of an atypical orgasm as by the absence of one, as we will see in Chapter 13, "Sexuality and Personal Evolution". These states are close to mystic ecstasy. Sexuality and religion have more in common than those who are religious generally intend. The English novelist, D. H. Lawrence, the author of *Lady Chatterley's Lover*, exalts sexuality as a means of attaining truth and fulfillment. The American writer, Henry Miller, author of the *Sexus*, *Plexus* and *Nexus* trilogy, sees sex as a possibility for inner freedom. Perhaps it is for this reason that these authors were prohibited in many countries for years.

These observations follow from the concept, referred to at the beginning of the chapter, that layers of environmental influence – the personality – develop around a vital energetic nucleus – the essence. In critical (climax) situations of intense pain, danger, or pleasure, the personality is momentarily diluted, allowing for re-contact with one's essence. It is a kind of instantaneous "death" of the personality, of the psychological identity. At this moment, the dialectic of opposites, death/life, comes to the fore.

References

Costa, R. P. (1994). *Os onze sexos – As múltiplas faces da sexualidade humana (The eleven sexes – The multiple faces of human sexuality)*. São Paulo: Gente.

Ferreira-Santos, E. (1996). *O ciúme, o medo da perda (Jealousy, the fear of loss)*. São Paulo, Ática.

Fonseca, J. (1980). *Psicodrama da loucura (The psychodrama of madness)*. São Paulo: Ágora.

Klein, M. (1996). *Amor, culpa e reparação e outros trabalhos (1921–1945)*. Rio de Janeiro: Imago. (Original edition: *Love, guilt and reparation and other works*. London: The Melanie Klein Trust, 1975.)

Kohut, H. (1984). *Self e narcisismo*. Rio de Janeiro: Zahar Editores S.A. (Original edition: *The search for the self – selected writings of Heinz Kohut: 1950–1978* (2 vols). New York: International Universities Press, Inc., 1978.)

Miller, H. (1974). *O mundo do sexo*. Rio de Janeiro: Companhia Editora Americana. (Original edition: *The world of sex*. Chicago: Argus Book Shop, 1941.)

Moreno, J. L. (1961). *Psicodrama*. Buenos Aires: Hormé. (Original edition: *Psychodrama – First Volume*. New York: Beacon House, Inc., 1946.)

---

5 Tiba (1986) analyses the sexual encounter according to the Rojas-Bermudez "nucleus of I" theory.

Moreno, J. L. (1977) *Psychodrama – First Volume* (5th edn). New York: Beacon House, Inc.

Moreno, J. L. (1993). *Psicodrama*. São Paulo: Cultrix. (Original edition: *Psychodrama – First Volume*. New York: Beacon House, Inc., 1946.)

Perazzo, S. (1986) *Descansem em paz os nossos mortos dentro de mim (May those who have died rest in peace inside me)*. Rio de Janeiro: Francisco Alves.

Tiba, I. (1986). *Puberdade e adolescência: desenvolvimento biopsicossocial (Puberty and adolescence: bio-psychosocial development)*. São Paulo: Ágora.

Wechsler, M. P. F. (1997). A matriz de identidade numa perspectiva construtivista: locus de construção de conhecimento (The matrix of identity from a constructivist perspective: locus of the construction of knowledge). *Revista Brasileira de Psicodrama*, 5, 1: 21–28.

Williams, A. (1994). *Psicodrama estratégico*. São Paulo: Ágora. (Original edition: *The passionate technique – Strategic Psychodrama with individuals, families and groups*. London: Routledge, 1989.)

Chapter 11

Sexual identity

Existential identity, sexual identity and relational sexual identity[1]

According to Greenson (1982), heterosexual identity formation can be summarized to three basic points. Take the example of a boy who recognizes:

1   I am John, a person.
2   I am John, a little boy.
3   I am John, a little boy, which means that I like to do sexual things with girls.

The way in which an individual experiences these points results in his/her adult sexual definition. In the *indifferentiation* or *symbiosis* or *double* phase, boys are *mixed* with a woman, the mother. Supposedly, marks of this double identity, feminine–masculine, remain. Am I a man or a woman? Or, how much woman am I? These are common fears in childhood and adolescence. Men, more commonly than women, are afraid and angry about being identified as homosexuals, which means having feminine aspects. A woman, from this perspective, should get her sexual identity more easily: she is separated from a woman (mother) and learns how to be one from this same woman; that is, she begins the *recognition of the sexual I* with her own mother. As Winnicott (1975) says, the feminine *is* while the masculine *is made*. Greenson (1982) refers to this possibility to justify that the majority of doubts about sexual identity reside in men. This fact is corroborated by the considerably greater number of men who seek sex-change surgeries. In the same way, there are an indisputably greater number of male transvestites and transexuals than female ones.

---

1 Consult the book by Ronaldo Pamplona da Costa (1994), *The eleven sexes* (heterosexual women, heterosexual men, homosexual men, lesbian women, bisexual men, transvestites, transsexuals and hermaphrodites). Also consult *Masculine/feminine* by Luiz Cushnir (1992).

The negative imprints of the *recognition of the sexual I* and the *ideal sexual I* phases are manifested by insecurity and doubt about the body as a whole and the genitals in particular. Concerns abut penis size, for example, are entirely common in our culture. Performance anxiety, both for men as well as women, is another example. How much man (or woman) am I?

From a didactic point of view, *the recognition of the sexual you* phase promotes sexual knowledge of people of the opposite sex. *Not knowing* (the sex of) the other brings out anxiety that varies according to the characteristics of the other person and the type of relationship established. A new loving relationship always brings on a certain degree of anxiety that dissolves as time passes, or when there is a better *role reversal*. Men *fear/ desire* women, and vice versa. Just as women admire–envy the penis, men admire–envy a women's ability to bear children.

Utilizing and going further with the identity formation scheme, let us speculate on the way that an individual establishes homosexual patterns. The examples will be of men, since my clinical experience is considerably greater with male homosexuals.

In this case, then, the three points would be:

1   I am John, a person.
2   I am John, a boy.
3   I am John, who, despite being a boy, likes to do sexual things with boys.

There is, therefore, in relation to heterosexuals, a difference only with the third point, since the male homosexual accepts his sexual identity as male. His relational sexual identity, however, is directed toward people of the same sex.

With transexuals, the following is observed:

1   I am John, a person.
2   I am John, who, despite being a boy, would like to be a girl (Joanna).
3   I am John, who, despite being a boy, would like to be a girl (Joanna) and likes to do sexual things with boys.

In this case, there are differences in points 2 and 3. The nuclear identity (I am a person named John, despite not agreeing with this) remains preserved. These people seek a female identity through hormonal treatments, plastic surgery and changing their male names for female ones.

Point 1 is altered in existential identity disorders, when the individual is confused about his existence in the world: who am I? do I exist? These clinical patterns are manifested in different identity disorder syndromes and psychotics.

Homosexuality

Observation of the *masculine homosexual manifestation* reveals, first of all, that its presentation comes in many forms, such as the sexual preference of being active or passive. Second, one notes that some psychodynamics recur among these people. In psychodramatic language, one could say that the primary social atom (primary sociometry), or *matrix of identity*, of homosexuals contains some patterns. However, it cannot be stated that this is characteristic of homosexuality, as it is also found in families of heterosexuals. Good sense suggests that a sufficiently attractive male sexual model should be available for him *to learn* to be a man. Identified as being of the male gender, the individual initiates the relational process with women and perceives what he feels for them. What type of attraction, curiosity and pleasure does he have or not have for them? Do they generate fear? What type of fear?

It is common to find male homosexuals who present a persistent transferential connection with their mothers, and vice versa, demonstrating that their mothers are equally confused about their identity in relation to their sons. The mother who feels hatred, conscious or unconscious, toward men and, as a consequence, toward the father of her son, ends up complicating the boy's communication with his father, thereby frustrating the possibility of imitation and masculine identification. When, for whatever reason, the father really is absent, fragile or weak in his psychological and social structure, he lacks the power to attract his son to love and admire him. This conflict is further aggravated when the father presents relational difficulties with male figures and rejects the son. For such a boy, all that remains is to stay within the maternal territory, femininity, and, sometimes, homosexuality.

As has already been stated, this psychodynamic contains subtle relational gradations, appearing as much in homosexuals as in heterosexuals. There are, for example, men with obviously feminine personality traits who are not homosexual. A boy's necessity to admire his father, to love a man, may be transformed into hatred when it is frustrated. For example, one patient relives a childhood scene in which he tries to show his manual dexterity to his father (searching for the father's love), by proposing to fix a household appliance. The father disregards the child's capacity and ignores him. In the psychodramatic scene, the boy explodes with sadness and hatred. The *emptiness of men* remains to be filled during his life. Childhood and adolescent masculine idols present characters to identify with. In the homosexual, the admiration of the idol is consciously sexualized. One patient relates that during his adolescence he tried to maintain relations with older men who gave him money, even though he didn't have financial problems. He solidifies the psychodramatic scene with a symbolic image in which he appears sad, with his shoulders hunched. An older man comes from behind, takes him by the shoulders, places his knee on his buttocks, leaving him in an erect position, his chest open, more "manly". Symbolically, the older man injects masculinity in the youth.

It is observed in the psychotherapeutic clinic for homosexuals that there is a mirrored search for the idealized masculine image. Sometimes the homosexual searches for his own lost image in his partner. The search is reflective; he tries to complete himself in something that feels incomplete. One patient desired "the Marlboro man" (reference to a cigarette advertisement where a masculine cowboy is featured). This man of his dreams must be heterosexual. With humor, he added that if the cowboy wanted to have sex with him, the thrill would be lost, as he would be demonstrating homosexuality. This same patient hated gay nightclubs and environments and couldn't tolerate "flaming" gays.

In active as well as passive sexual practices, the homosexual finds himself in a narcissistic search for his lost or unfulfilled self-image. If the passive homosexual wants to receive a man inside himself, the active homosexual is satisfied by supposedly being "more man" than the other. Within this dynamic, the comparative–competitive expression between the partners is transparent.

The agonizing search for the sexual self-image may be manifested by compulsive or sadomasochistic homosexual practices. One patient reports that when he feels "crazy" for sex, he directs himself to public rest rooms where he engages in a variety of sexual acts (especially fellatio) with successive partners. After several hours, he feels relieved on the one hand, but dirty and guilty on the other. Another patient says that when he is "consumed" by sexual desire, he looks for, preferably, soldiers, blacks and blue-collar workers (for him, masculine stereotypes). After the sexual relations, he feels hatred for his partners, humiliating them because of their economic and social class. Clinically, a gradation of anxiety in the search for the *other's* masculinity is observed. This gradation reveals the degree of *love–jealousy–hatred* involved in the process. It can be summarized in four levels: *to receive, take, steal* and *rip out* the other's masculinity.[2] The last two clinical examples reveal moments of desperate sexual necessity, which are transformed into uncontrolled action. If the pathological manifestation reveals the extremity of the type, the examples are valid for reflection on the *normal.*

The erotic interest of a woman may bring out a homosexual's phobic aspects, such as the fear of being swallowed, suffocated, or annihilated (fear of losing identity and returning to the phase of undifferentiated chaos, of symbiosis). His defense mechanisms may transform the phobic component into coldness, indifference or, on the contrary, a friendly alliance formed to

---

2 See "Roles and their modes" in Chapter 2, "Freud, Moreno and bossa nova".

neutralize the threat of a female sexual advance. In one psychodramatic scene, the protagonist divides women into two types: the saintly, pure woman and the lewd, whorish woman. Faced with the latter, who generates fear, he feels diminished as a man. The former is mocked or disregarded, since she doesn't appear to be a threat. In the role reversal, while playing the saint, the protagonist transforms her little by little until she has become as obscene as the other. The conclusion is that they are both shameless, cruel and challenging.

Gradations of sexuality

I suggest that there is a scale with different gradations and possibilities for sexual identity going from the transexuals, then the homosexuals, followed by bisexuals and lastly heterosexuals. Another scale, now in terms of male sexual function–dysfunction, shows, at one extreme, sexual impotence to various degrees, then premature ejaculation, delayed ejaculation and, lastly, satisfactory sexual performance. In women, following the same pattern, there is vaginismus (involuntary muscular contraction impeding penetration), dispareunia (recurring pain during the sex act), different levels of anorgasmia and satisfactory sexual performance.

This scale, having the idea of gradation or movement implicit, yields the question of health–illness. What is sick and what is healthy from a sexual point of view? Different levels of experiential quality during the evolutionary phases of the personality and sexuality determine a person's degree of *sexual health–illness*. The line between health and illness is tenuous; if it was an error of psychiatry to label all homosexuals as sick, as they were in the past, then it is also incorrect to say the contrary – that all homosexuals are healthy. It is important to understand that the definition of the sexual role in homosexuals or heterosexuals in itself doesn't allow one to determine his/her degree of pathology/health. There are pathological homosexual manifestations and pathological heterosexual manifestations. An accurate evaluation of a person's level of health–illness must include the study of his other roles and the observation of his personality as a whole.

Homosexuality, in principle, is a variation of the statistical norm. The homosexual portion of the population, in numerical terms, is considerably less than that of heterosexuals. The fact that homosexuals are a social minority engenders relational difficulties that, in turn, may become psychological overload. Aside from having to face the fact that, in general, minorities aren't respected by the majority, the homosexual mirrors the projection of fears, insecurities and doubts of the heterosexual majority. In this discussion, which in certain aspects is more sociological than psychological, it is good to remember that homosexuality is not an option, as is commonly said, but rather an instinctive imposition. Sexual desire doesn't disappear with rational pondering, or with "good" advice. Sexual desire can be administrated, but not determined rationally. The only possible choice is either to restrain or liberate the heterosexual or homosexual impulse present, or sublimate it through sporting, artistic or religious activities.

A final consideration, not specific to homosexuality but including it, refers to the sexual development scheme presented here. The *ideal human being* would evolve perfectly through the phases described, like a god of sexual harmony and health. What would this individual be like? He would understand situations of love and rejection profoundly and spontaneously. He would have an excellent sexual identity (*recognition of the sexual I*) and an excellent perception of the opposite sex (*recognition of the sexual you*). He would resolve triangular situations without conflict, reverse roles freely, have the capacity to give himself wholly, and, free from muscular armor, would rise to the heavens with multiple orgasms.

Psychotherapy of homosexuals

In Chapter 4, "Personality Diagnosis and Identity Disorders", I divide psychotherapeutic patients, according to their different personality characteristics, into four groups: *normotics, neurotics, people with identity disorders* and *psychotics*. A study of the treatment of homosexuals in my private clinic reveals that, in relation to these groupings, they are distributed predominantly among the neurotics and those with sexual identity disorders. This data, however, doesn't necessarily reflect the social reality, much less mean that I have never attended psychotic or normotic homosexuals.

The psychotherapeutic process for homosexuals seeks the resolution of conflicts, among which are those referring to the existential, sexual and relational sexual identity formation. This would mean, in "surgical" terms, an operation of profound purpose. I don't customarily set a prior goal for psychotherapy; rather, I try to *discover the way, step by step*. However, if I were asked to synthesize some of the steps in the psychotherapy process for homosexuals, I would say that an important point is the *exorcism* of the paternal–maternal figures. I mean by *exorcism* that it isn't enough to understand (forgive) the conflicts, it is necessary to (re)live them in their three sociometric poles (attraction, neutrality and rejection). The problem isn't in the mother, the father, or the child. The question belongs to the relational network established in the past and which remains alive (untransformed) within the patient. Psychodrama is a valuable technique in this sense, as it helps the protagonist play both the father and mother he had and those he would like to have had. When he is able to reorganize this internal sociometry, which is also worked through in its tele–transferential (love–hate) aspects with the therapist, the patient is freed from the old scripts that imprisoned him. This can mean either the possibility for heterosexual experiences, formerly disregarded, or a more harmonious redimensioning of his homosexual life.

References

Costa, R. P. (1994). *Os onze sexos: as múltiplas faces da sexualidade humana (The eleven sexes: the multiple faces of human sexuality)*. São Paulo: Gente.

Cuschnir, L. (1992). *Masculino/feminina (Masculine/feminine)*. Rio de Janeiro: Rosa dos Tempos.

Echenique, M. and Fassa, M. E. G. (1992). *Poder e amor: a micropolítica das relações (Power and love: the micropolitics of relationships)*. São Paulo: Aleph.

Greenson, R. R. (1982). Um menino transexual e uma hipótese (A transexual boy and a hypothesis). In: *Investigações em psicanálise*), vol. 2. Rio de Janeiro: Imago. (Original edition: *Explorations in psychoanalysis*. New York: International Universities Press, Inc., 1978.)

Merengué, D. (1999). Sexualidades e espontaneidade criadora (Sexualities and creative spontaneity). *Revista Brasileira de Psicodrama (Brazilian Journal of Psychodrama)*, 7, 2.

Stoller, R. (1993). *Masculinidade e feminilidade (Masculinity and femininity)*. Porto Alegre: Artes Médicas.

Winnicott, D. W. (1975). *O brincar e a realidade*. Rio de Janeiro: Imago. (Original edition: *Playing and reality*. London: Tavistock Publications Ltd., 1971.)

Chapter 12

Sexual sociometry and forms of sexuality

A boy loved a maiden, but she preferred another, who another maiden loved.

Heinrich Heine*

The sociometry[1] of sex follows from Moreno's (1978) assertions regarding the possibilities for interpersonal relationships: attraction, rejection and neutrality (*ne uter*, in Latin, which is neither one nor the other), or indifference.

Sociometric choice within a group of people is always based on some criteria. For example, if the criteria is to study, the options will be: whom I choose (positive) to study with me, whom I don't choose (negative) and whom I am indifferent or neutral toward. A common criterion permits, from the explicit reciprocal choices of the members, the study of the apparent and concealed networks of group sociodynamics. If the criteria is sexual attraction, those who attract positively, those who do not attract, and those who cause indifference come into the network of multiple and complex interactions. From the result, one knows who chooses whom, to what extent the choices are *congruent* or *incongruent* and what the situation (value) of the individual is within the group in terms of sexual attractiveness. Taking this *sociometric test* even further, the individual's capacity to perceive how many times he/she will be chosen is also measured. This *perceptual test* gives the individual's *telic* capacity index. In an extreme illustration, a person may believe that he/she will receive all the positive choices and actually get none, and vice versa.

Sexual attraction is intrinsic to humans. A gathering of people – in the classroom, subway, church or therapeutic group – is enough to ignite it.

---

* Apud Ouspensky (1980), p. 561.
1 Sociometry is the method created by J. L. Moreno by which he proposes to study and measure relational interactions within a group.

Sexual antennae are always turned on, even when one isn't in the mood for or consciously deliberating about the search for a sexual encounter.

There are types of people who provoke sexual desire (positive), neutral types, and repulsive types (negative). Sexual desire rests in biological, psychological and sociocultural dimensions. For some, there is even a cosmic dimension in the processes of loving and sexual choices.

Ouspensky (1961) states that an individual feels one of four types of attraction toward another person and vice versa. The first type of attraction is for the rare people who are irresistible. These people always remain new and unknown. There are elements of fascination and magic in these relationships. Type two people inspire a more tranquil attraction, which fits into the conventional shape of loving relationships. The feeling of love may change to friendship or even diminish or disappear, but a thankful, sweet memory always remains. Type three people inspire indifference. When they are young and attractive they may affect, at times, a sexual fantasy, but this attraction soon disappears. The first sexual encounter usually extinguishes whatever sexual flame there was. The persistence of the relationship may generate ill-will or hostility. Type four people cause repugnance. Sexual relations with this type of person usually contain some tragic element, given the opposition to sex inherent to the situation. The continuation of the relationship becomes a violation of individuality that can lead to *inferior* sexuality.

Ancient history reveals that the marriage sacrament was performed by someone (a priest) adept at perceiving the sexual types of the two proposing to get married. In accordance with his knowledge and experience he would make a recommendation on the union. This would later become the marriage rite officiated by a priest.

The idea that sexual types mutually gravitate is part of the allegory of two separate halves (of the man and woman) who seek each other. It is said that on Olympus, one god stood out for his uncommon beauty, provoking envy in the other gods. The envy was so great that the god wound up splitting down the middle. The two halves were the origins of man and woman. And when they meet in love a divine spark is ignited.

From a psychodramatic point of view, the mutual gravitation of sexual types is revealed in accordance with the *telic–transferential* possibilities. *Telic–transferential* choices contain both a conscious and unconscious component. *Telic* loving relationships are characterized by the acuity of the reciprocal choices. Transferential choices are found in erroneous relationships and distorted perceptions; for example, a relationship composed of a type 1 man and a type 4 woman, or vice versa. Different transferential combinations can occur. As shown, the most harmonious couplings are formed by combining types 1 and 2 – that is, a type 1 man with a type 1 woman; a type 2 man with a type 2 woman; a type 1 man with a type 2 woman; or a type 2 man with a type 1 woman.

Another aspect to be considered refers to the duration of the gravitational forces of sexual attraction. Just as passion is a phase, the level of sexual attraction between partners is a cycle of polarities that is transformed over time. This means that couples may oscillate between types of attraction (from 1 to 4) during the relationship. Administrating these variations, including maintaining or terminating the relationship, and submitting to or opposing family or cultural pressures, signifies, perhaps, a wisdom that few couples reach.[2]

Forms of sexuality

Reciprocal attraction in sexual pairs is one of the main life forces. The intensity and quality of its manifestations determine important personal characteristics. A healthy human presents an explicit attraction for sex. Many times, the first symptom of a physical or psychological disease is the loss of this attraction, though, since extremes are closely connected, an exaggerated interest in sex is also observed in some health alterations. The more intellectually and emotionally rich a person is, the higher his comprehension of sex will be. The beauty of the sex act connects sexuality to aesthetics. Eroticism, sensuality and art are interconnected.

Nature created more sexual attraction in humans than is necessary for the purpose of preserving the species. This *excess* may take positive or negative directions. Freud (1968) speaks of *sublimating* the libido through art. Some ancient religious systems also make reference to the transmutation of sexual energy in terms of spiritual evolution. Others preach the ritual exercise of sexuality oriented toward consciousness development. Moralism and repression would be negative ways of dealing with sexual energy. The positive forms of directing sexuality are under the protection of *fluency* while the negative forms are under the tyranny of reclusion.

Superior, normal and inferior sexuality

According to Ouspensky (1961), sexuality can be divided into three categories: *inferior sexuality*, *normal sexuality* and *superior sexuality*. *Inferior sexuality* is manifested either explicitly or implicitly. It is found in criminal behavior, licentiousness and unhealthy moralism. *Inferior sexuality* is found in the rituals of religious sects with low spirituality. Any manifestation that degrades sex belongs to *inferior sexuality*. While sex may by joyful, it is far from comical. Pornography, which disrespects the sex act, is included in *inferior sexuality*. There is a difference between pornography and erotic art.

---

2 See *The loving link: the path of affective life*, by Luiza Ricotta (1994).

While the former ridicules, the latter exalts the poetry of loving movement. *Inferior sexuality* drains psychic energy; the person who practices it becomes exhausted. In *normal sexuality*, on the other hand, the psychic energy employed is recovered, due to the positive nature of the sensations, thoughts and emotions involved. After *normal sex*, the person feels reinvigorated and happy, not empty and melancholy.

It is a characteristic of humans (and some other species) to demonstrate affection and sexual excitement through squeezing, embracing, kissing and biting. Sadomasochistic elements are inherent to love and sex. Sadomasochistic demonstrations may represent either a healthy manifestation (superior or normal sexuality) or a pathological one, belonging to *inferior sexuality*. What distinguishes the two is the energy taken away. The former is constructive, connected to life; the latter is destructive, linked to death. In sexual crimes there is a pathological dimension to the sadomasochistic releases. Killing is not enough; it is also necessary to torture with cold-blooded perversity.

In ancient religious doctrines, the higher purpose of sexuality was the possibility of spiritual birth or growth. The scholastic and ecclesiastic religions, such as Buddhism, Judaism, Christianity and Islamism, feared the appeal that the practices of *superior sexuality* might have to the people. So they abolished the category of *superior sexuality* that deals with the transmutation of sexual energy through the practice of sex. They maintained, however, a category that proposes the transmutation of sexual energy to spiritual energy through sexual abstinence. Only the absence of sexual practices would elevate one to God.

Judean-Christian philosophy, with its pleasure–guilt dyad, created sex-guilt or sex-sin. However, some ancient religions, prior to the onset of these values, considered sexuality a divine expression and, therefore, the object of adoration. Many expressions along these lines are found in the ancient religions of Greece, Rome, Crete, Egypt and India. Their religious sculptures show erotic phalluses, images and ceremonial dances. Tantric philosophy is based on reliving the union of the cosmic couple, Shiva and Shakti. Shiva is the masculine principle, symbol of transcendental power, and Shakti is the feminine energy, the intuitive representation of wisdom.

Regression and reversion

Some authors believe that a libidinal regression occurs during the sex act. They add that, under these circumstances, the oral, anal and genital phases of psychological development are relived. It is true that sexual excitation is manifested by well-noted physiological changes, such as rapid breathing, dilatation of the pupils, peripheral vasodilatation and intumescence and lubrication of the sexual organs. That is, there is erotic sensitivity throughout the body, especially in the erogenous zones. One cannot say, however, that there is a simple regression. The *quality* of adult sexual excitation is different from the libidinal state of the first phases of sexual development, if only because one occurs in childhood and the other in adulthood. Reliving these zones in *normal* and *super-sexuality* has a different *quality* than that of childhood. In both *childhood play* and adult *sex games* there is ludic behavior that reflects spontaneity, pleasure and living in the moment. But I don't believe these characteristics can necessarily be called regressive. During sexual relations (unconscious) narcissistic reminiscences come into play in which the person feels he is the most beautiful and unique, the greatest. In pathological sexuality (*inferior sexuality*), the narcissistic reminiscences are frustrating, depressing and aggressive.

As a way of classifying these sexual manifestations, I propose utilizing the concepts of *regression* and *reversion*.[3] *Regression's* polar opposite is progress. *Regression–progression* is defined by a disorderly movement in the direction of something or some place. For example, São Paulo is cited as a city of great *progress*, although its growth has been disorganized and chaotic. Or, when someone has had a "psychotic *regression*", what is meant is that he/she began to present psychological patterns that were supposedly infantile and inappropriate for his/her age. *Reversion's* polar opposite is *process*. *Reversion–process* is delineated by organized, harmonious movement. *Regression* and *reversion* both turn backward, but present completely different organizational qualities. *Progress* and *process* move forward, but also with distinct structural qualities.

Regression is a return to the old organizational patterns, to an untransformed past. It belongs to the *transferential* world. Reversion, though it has connections to the past, has a present organizational pattern, superior to the previous stage. It is in the *tele* world. Therefore, reversion is part of the evolutionary process in a being who grows. In reversion, the past is transformed. *Normal* and *superior sexuality* possess *reversive* structures. *Inferior sexuality* contains a *regressive* structure.

References

Freud, S. (1968). "Analisis fragmentario de una histeria (Caso Dora)". *Obras Completas*, vol. II. Madrid: Editorial Biblioteca Nueva, pp. 605–658. (English edition: *Fragment of an analysis of a case of hysteria (Dora's Case)*. Complete psychological works of Sigmund Freud, vol. VII, pp. 51–52. London: Hogarth Press, 1905.)

Laing, R. (1978). Aulas e supervisões proferidas na FMUSP, São Paulo (Classes and supervisions given at the School of Medicine at the University of São Paulo).

3 See Laing (1978).

Moreno, J. L. (1978). *Who shall survive? – Foundations of sociometry, group psychotherapy and sociodrama.* New York: Beacon House, Inc.

Ouspensky, P. D. (1980). *Un nuevo modelo del universo.* Buenos Aires: Hormé (English edition: *A new model of the universe.* London: Routledge and Kegan Paul, 1961.)

Ricotta, L. C. A. (1994). *O vínculo amoroso: a trajetória da vida afetiva (The loving link: the path of affective life).* São Paulo: Iglu.

Chapter 13

Sexuality and personal evolution*

I thought a lot about how to develop this theme in a clear and objective way. To approach it theoretically I would have had to consult a great deal of literature on the subject, which deviates from my current proposal. So, I've resolved to do this by way of a clinical report.

Some years ago, I treated a 35-year-old man psychotherapeutically for one year. He lived in a distant city which meant that he could only come to the sessions every two weeks, and at times just once a month. I accepted his suggestion that he write to me between consultations. Ten years later, I saw him again to focus on another problem. Upon his return, we went over many of the episodes that had occurred at the time of his earlier treatment. He was then able to clarify, probably more for me than for him, some of the shady points of his strange experiences. Based on this information, with his permission and with literary license, I will reconstruct his case.

Although he was young, he had been married for ten years and had three children. He married his high-school girlfriend whom he had dated throughout his adolescence. He presented an obsessive-phobic personality structure. He did not present, however, symptoms corresponding to this type of psychological structure; that is, he had neither obsessive nor phobic complaints. I considered him normotic (see Chapter 4, "Personality Diagnosis and Identity Disorders"). He was a talented young man who easily distinguished himself professionally as an executive of a large business. He had always been shy with women. He confessed to having been faithful to his wife more as a result of his timidness than his determination. Nevertheless, he had initiated a romance with a married woman and was worried about the consequences of the new relationship. To his surprise, he didn't feel guilty. His self-esteem increased as his lover, described as very attractive and experienced, praised his sexual performance. He seemed almost childishly happy about being approved by an adult woman. In this sense, his wife was the woman–child coupled with the man–boy.

* Work presented at the São Paulo Psychodrama Society in November of 1992.

The sexual encounters at first took place in motels. But, concerned that they would be recognized on the way, they finally found refuge in a safe place. These moments represented "an island of peace" from the confusion of their lives.

The encounters, initially characterized by strong sensuality, later began to follow another sequence. As soon as they arrived, they bathed, ate, drank wine and occasionally smoked marijuana. Caresses were intermingled with long conversations, which sometimes lasted hours. In this way, sexual excitement was maintained at a plateau for long periods. Bit by bit, the conversation would diminish and the bodily dialogue increase. In silence, they would touch and explore each other sensually. The penetration phase is described as different from earlier experiences:

> My whole body moved in waves. I thought that my movements were feminine, but I didn't mind. I wanted to discover myself, to know myself. I began losing my fear of myself and realized that I was also becoming less afraid of life. Until then, I had considered myself sexually experienced, but it was really summed up by a few experiences with prostitutes and my wife. I realized how timid I'd been in bed. I dared to exploit the intimacy of my girlfriend's body and, surprisingly, she liked it. I had had a puritanical view of women. But, if someone had said this to me before, I would have been offended.

His orgasms became longer and more pleasurable. When he was very young, he'd had manifestations of premature ejaculation that diminished after marrying. He correlated these episodes to anxious situations. During his first meetings with his lover, worried about his sexual performance, they occurred again.

Another passage from our protagonist:

> As the months passed, I observed a great modification in my way of relating sexually. I became less and less concerned about the final orgasm. I began to enjoy the details of the sensations. For example, from a visual point of view, I became enchanted with the curves of her body. I realized that different visualizations were possible, depending on whether my eyes were closer or further away or open or partially closed. I discovered details of forms and movements. I observed the intersection of lines and contrasts between light and dark. Shadow and light gained new meaning. I, who had never been interested in art, began to admire paintings. I even bought the fascicles of a collection of great painters. All of my senses developed, especially smell, touch and sight. Everything was calmer and more intense. But the most memorable experience occurred a few months later. We had talked and aroused each other quite a bit. During the whole time, I remained

inside her, without movement (I frequently leaned against the head of the bed in a way that I was half sitting, half lying and she stayed on top). Then light waves began to run through my solar plexus. I realized that something similar was also happening with her. We abandoned ourselves and let it happen. The waves began slowly increasing. We stayed this way for a long time, in total silence, but completely conscious. I experienced a succession of sensations. It was as if I were divided in two: one who felt and another who observed. It was as if there were a couple in the bed and I was hovering above them observing. At some point I had the feeling that we were levitating. I was never a spiritist, and to tell the truth, never really liked these things, but I had the feeling that something very different was happening. At some point I began to see lights, colors and shapes. Everything was very clear. It is difficult to express in words. I wasn't sure who was I and who was she; it was as if we were one. It was as if I didn't have a name. I was me and not me at the same time. But this didn't upset me; on the contrary, it brought me peace. It was as if I were alive and dead at the same time. "Death", which had always frightened me, was experienced in peace. On television, I've heard the statements of people who had near-death experiences. What I experienced was very similar to this. In short, after an undefined period (time is a way of speaking, since time didn't exist), I began to sense that I was having an orgasm, but it wasn't a common orgasm. I felt a bluish energy coming from me at the same time that my head was bathed in a clear, bright light. My whole body vibrated. Slowly we came back to earth. We stayed inside each other, quietly hugging. She began crying softly. She said they were tears of longing. I didn't ask any questions because I understood . . .

Initially, he had had the tendency to overvalue the importance of his lover in the experience. However, she didn't give him the sensations, nor did he give them to her. They both experienced a special moment, *through* each other. The *through* is essential in understanding that no one gives pleasure to anyone. Pleasure is had *through* the other. There is no place for greater or less, nor for better or worse. Each is responsible for his or her own pleasure. The *other* is the catalyst of our own pleasure. The sexual partners are co-responsible. By responsibility I mean the capacity and discernment to respond to internal and external stimuli, containing or liberating them.

In the days that followed, our protagonist was in a state of exaltation. He felt strong and courageous. He went to bed late and woke up early. He began to take initiatives that before he had lacked the courage to undertake. I feared that he was entering a state of hypomania. Psychiatric training forms and sometimes deforms, in the sense of unduly "pathologizing" emotional states. Fortunately, I was able to realize that it wasn't a case of pathological exaltation of the mood. He showed himself to be confident, full of ideas and projects. He felt happy and secure. Many things began to change in his life. The romance with the lover continued. But, what will come as a surprise and disappointment to some, he felt encouraged to meet other women.

What happened then was what he called "a return to the past": he maintained relationships with women he had desired in his youth but hadn't had the courage to approach at the time. He decided to separate from his wife, which made him feel very guilty. But this guilt, which before had paralyzed him, no longer impeded him from making decisions. He quit his job and started his own business. He experienced the sensation of being true to himself and to others. He hid nothing from his lover, who accompanied, astonished, these transformations in his life. His relatives thought he had gone mad. His parents told him he was throwing away the security of his family and job. His male friends told him it wasn't necessary to get separated in order to have affairs. Some couples distanced themselves; others opted to stay friends with his ex-wife. The wives of his friends considered him a "bad example". In short, as with all revolutions, be they personal, social or political, powerful forces of repression had to be faced. He thought about moving to another city, but his strong connection to his children prevented him. His lover, probably shocked by the changes in him, resolved to "invest" in her own marriage and ended the relationship. He felt lonely and sad, but after a while got through the phase. A new life announced itself; everything was about to happen. He had several girl-friends, his business prospered, some of his old friends returned, other new ones were made. Years later, he married again. He found a happy and harmonious relationship. But that is another story, for another time.

I would like to reflect on some of the points this man experienced. In the first place, the fact that he sought therapeutic help when he was in the middle of a growth process (or crisis) calls attention. This is inferred from the fact that he began the psychotherapy after he had already begun the relationship with his lover. As I have observed many times, some people intuitively sense that a phase of transformation is about to occur. In this situation, the psychotherapist is invited more to follow along than to intervene in the process. Another question is how much the sexual experience itself was relevant. That is, were the sexual experiences determining factors or consequences of the personal transformation process? It is fitting to make a distinction between *change* and *transformation*. *Change* means the natural alterations of life, natural results of the passage of time. No effort is necessary; it happens by itself. *Transformation*, on the other hand, requires intention, a conscious and deliberate effort focused on internal growth. If both processes were propelled by energy, *transformation* would consume a more refined fuel. When our protagonist put together his energy to consciously transgress, from a personal and socio-familiar point of view, he was already in the process of transformation. From a psychodynamic point of view, one could say that the obsessive-phobic structure became more flexible, permitting the liberation of the imprisoned affective and sexual content. There was an impulse of health and growth. The *I observer* developed, as is described symbolically in our character's own report, when he sees himself "observed by himself". In this sense, the crisis experienced gains the connotation of *healthy craziness*. This assertion is reminiscent of the anti-psychiatry of the 1960s and 1970s which understood insanity as an attempt at self-healing. It is reminiscent, as well, of the *similia similibus curantur* of homeopathic medicine – in this case, insanity curing insanity.

A tantric reading of the experience permits a series of correlations. Tantrism is a broad oriental philosophy that proposes the sexual rite as one of the paths to transcendence. In tantric sexual practice, the partners deliberately try to experience an altered state of mystical consciousness. They seek the union of masculine and feminine characteristics; that is, the harmony of opposites in the sense of reaching totality. When the opposites are liberated, the partners gain wholeness. Polar opposites aren't contradictions but rather complements. In the tantric tradition, the fusion of the feminine–masculine contains a sacred dimension, as if God were present. Tantric sexual practice recommends choosing an appropriate place, where the partners won't be interrupted from their mutual devotion, a ritual bath, the utilization of aromatic oils and a meal (composed of aphrodisiac foods) with wine (some rituals prescribe the ingestion of other drugs). Foreplay receives special attention, performed with the focus of sensorial attention. This procedure permits the delay or inexistence of physical orgasm. In this way, there would be a flow of sexual energy to the superior centers and the possibility of ecstasy. I believe that the experience reported here has some correlation to this description.

From the point of view of the roles involved in the experience, one can see that there was a development of the sexual and social roles – professional as well as familiar. The roles of lover, son, husband, father and executive suffered profound transformations. This meant breaking from the past and gaining a new perspective on the future. These observations reinforce Moreno's (1977) and Bustos's (1999) affirmations on role *clusters*: there is communication among roles with the possibility of mutual benefit. From a psychodramatic point of view, the events can be interpreted as a *catharsis of integration* in the life scene, to the extent that our protagonist put out (*das ding ausser sich*)[1] his internal world and, from that point on, fostered its reorganization, with the respective consequences in his social life.

According to the observations concerning the development of sexuality discussed in Chapter 10, "Sexuality as a Relational Instrument", one can

1 Consult "The protagonic state of being outside oneself: some notes" (Merengué, 1994).

understand that our protagonist's experience is inserted in the context of the sexual *encounter*. This can be synthesized as a spontaneous experience of role reversal between the participants, loss and fusion of identities, momentary dissolution of the personality (depersonalization) and contact with the essence, sensation of life–death (*little death*), escape from chronological time and experience of *eternal time*. The register of an inexpressible moment remains.

In accordance with Chapter 12, "Sexual Sociometry and Forms of Sexuality", the experience related here belongs to *superior sexuality*. As was commented, loving and mystic experiences have some similarities. Amorous and mystic ecstasy both release the same type of energy or, in other words, present a similar experiential quality. Anand (1992) states that, from questionnaires and interviews, <u>she</u> (and not he) determined that sex may lead to mystical or sacred experiences. She adds that "sacred sex", the experience of ecstasy, may be the basis for a new sexual revolution.

Jung (1989) studies, in *Mysterium Coniunctionis*, the alchemic conception of the union of opposites. Alchemists intended, through the union (*coniunctio*) of substances, to reach a greater objective; that is, the production of gold. The materials, man and woman, can be transformed into spiritual gold by means of a mysterious method (*Non fieri transitum nisi per medium* – passage doesn't occur without a means).

Ecstasy mobilizes the superior centers of the personality (the superior emotional and intellectual centers. See Chapter 6, "Internal Psychodrama"). From a physiological point of view, biochemical reactions are responsible for the inhibition–liberation of neurotransmitters responsible for the extraordinary feelings experienced. Modern psychopharmacology should concern itself not only with pathological manifestations (hallucinations, *delirium*), but also with the states of sexual and mystical ecstasy.

The sexual climax (*peak experience*) described is one of man's grandiose experiences. These are comprised of situations that transcend the quotidian, experienced within the narcissistic context of the personality. They are correlated to the *ideal sexual I* described in Chapter 10, "Sexuality as a Relational Instrument". In this case, they constitute healthy narcissistic experiences of fluency and harmony. The approximation of these states with Moreno's (1977) spontaneity–creativity is inevitable. For him, the first characteristic of a creative act is its spontaneity. The second is the sensation of surprise, of something unexpected. The third is the sense of unreality, to the extent that the causal nexus of the life process is broken. The fourth characteristic is the transformation of the *sui generis* of the patient to the agent; that is, the feature that distinguishes the creature from the creator. The fifth characteristic of the creative act is to produce imitation effects. For Moreno, man's creative acts incorporate God.

The states of consciousness experienced by the patient during the culminating moments can be understood as *altered states of consciousness*.

Here, mystical and religious trances – for example, those of the Evangelical and Afro-Brazilian sects[2] – would also be included. As a psychiatrist, I have been able to follow clinically some psychotic profiles unleashed by these types of trances. People with a weak personality structure present difficulty in containing and elaborating the experience. Fortunately, this was not the case with our protagonist, who utilized it as a growth factor. This type of experience resembles certain drugs that, depending on the dosage, can act as either medicine or poison, curing or killing.

Love–sex is situated in the relational sphere. Relationship–separation is connected to life–death, beginning–end. Sexuality, love and relationships are within the *I–you* orbit and in the search for the *eternal you* (God) about which Martin Buber, the relationship philosopher, speaks.

The fascination which sexuality incites is connected to love in a broad sense. The union of man and woman was consolidated as a path to the absolute: "in God, neither woman is independent from man, nor man independent from woman" (I Corinthians, 11: 11). This "re-encounter" appears in all the great relational myths: in platonic love, the basis of the unique romance, in the myths of *Androgino*, in *Orpheus and Euridice*, in *Pygmalion and Galatea*, and in other myths found in all cultures throughout the ages.

References

Anand, M. (1992). *A arte do êxtase*. Rio de Janeiro: Campus. (Original edition: *The art of sexual ecstasy*. Los Angeles: Jeremy P. Tarcher, Inc., 1989.)

Bustos, D. (1999). *Novas cenas para o psicodrama. O teste da mirada e outros temas (New scenes for psychodrama. The* mirada *test and other themes)*. São Paulo: Ágora.

Jung, C. G. (1989). *Mysterium Coniunctionis*. Petrópolis: Vozes. (Original edition: *Mysterium Coniunctionis*. Olten: Walter-Verlag, 1971.)

Merengué, D. (1994). O estar fora de si protagtônico: algumas anotações (The protagonic state of being outside oneself: some notes). In: S. R. A. Petrilli, *Rosa-dos-ventos da teoria do psicodrama*. São Paulo: Ágora.

Moreno, J. L. (1977). *Psychodrama – First Volume* (5th edn). New York: Beacon House, Inc.

Motta, J. M. C. (1994). *Jogos: repetição ou criação? (Games: repetition or creation?)*. São Paulo, Plexus.

2 Merengué (1994) calls attention to the theatrical nature of the Catholic, Pentecostal and Afro-Brazilian rituals. Motta (1994) remembers the interaction of theater and religion during the Middle Ages.

Part 4

The past and future of psychodrama

Chapter 14

Moreno and the IAGP

The beginnings of the International Association of Group Psychotherapy*

After being elected to the IAGP Board of Directors, I became interested in promoting the organization in Brazil. So, I spoke with the organizers of the next Brazilian Congress of Psychodrama and asked for an opportunity to explain what the IAGP and its mission are. The organizers promptly arranged a place for me in a section of the Congress called "Speaking of . . ." Well, I had the space, so I needed the content, but I knew very little about the history of the IAGP.

At the next IAGP Board meeting, I happily communicated to our Secretary and to our President that I had found an important space to promote the organization in Brazil and that I needed information about the history of the IAGP. Initially they told me that we had some historical information on file, but I responded that I needed more. So the President suggested that I be the person to organize this data. I accepted the task and thus became a member of the Archives Committee (from 1995–1998). The following is the result of my work.

I began my research reading some texts about the beginnings of the IAGP in the few sources of literature available. I also wrote to people who had, in one way or another, participated in the origins of the organization, many of whom provided important information on the subject. At the International Congress of Group Psychotherapy, which took place in London in 1998, there was a day designated for interviews, discussions and round-tables with ex-presidents and ex-members of the Executive Committee. The IAGP also began to record interviews with key people in its history. In this way, additional information was gathered. Future researchers will have at their disposal, in addition to the Moreno Archives at Harvard University, new archives that are being organized under the supervision of René Marineau at the University of Trois Rivières (Canada) consisting of Anne Ancelin Schützenberger's personal library and files.

---

* J. Fonseca, The beginnings of IAGP: an historical approach, *The International Forum of Group Psychotherapy*, vol. 6, no. 2, 1997.

Moreno created a series of publications (journals and magazines) and associations throughout his career. He felt the need to organize the psychodramatic and the group psychotherapy movement. Moreno is credited with establishing the following organizations: the Society of Psychodrama and Group Psychotherapy in 1942, renamed the American Society of Group Psychotherapy and Psychodrama in 1951; the American Sociometric Association in 1945; and, what interests us particularly, the International Committee on Group Psychotherapy in Paris in 1951, the International Council of Group Psychotherapy in Milan in 1963, and, finally, the international incorporation of the IAGP in Zurich in 1973.

In fact, in his later years Moreno recognized that, more important than his battles – first with psychoanalysis, then with S. R. Slavson in terms of pioneering group psychotherapy – would be to have an organization where all the trends in group psychotherapy were represented.

With the end of the Second World War, international scientific meetings began to take place again. The First World Congress of Psychiatry was held in Paris in 1950. After this, psychotherapists felt prepared to have their own congresses, so in April of 1951 Moreno founded the International Committee of Group Psychotherapy, also in Paris. The objectives of the Committee (*Group Psychotherapy*, 1951, p. 126) were:

(1) to define the professional standards of group psychotherapy and to work towards a consensus of terms and operations; (2) to prepare for the international congresses; (3) to sponsor the International Archives of Group Psychotherapy.

Besides Moreno, other leaders of the group movement participated on the first Advisory Board: Foulkes (UK), Bierer (UK), Favez-Boutonier (France), Snowden (UK), P. Senft (UK), Delay (France), Heuyer (France), Lazelle (USA), Montassut (France), Porcher (France) and J.H. Pratt (USA). Zerka Moreno (1954, p. 91) notes:

The objective was a World Federation of Societies interested in group psychotherapy and allied subjects. Thanks to the combined efforts of Drs. W. Hulse, W. Warner, J. L. Moreno and S. R. Slavson, the International Committee on Group Psychotherapy took its present form, representing twenty-four countries.

The result of the formation of this Committee was the First International Congress of Group Psychotherapy in Toronto, Canada, in August of 1954, coincidentally the same city in which, in May of 1931 under the initiative of J. L. Moreno, the first organizing step on behalf of group psychotherapy was made during the meeting of the American Psychiatric Association. This was followed by the Round Table Conference on the Application of the

Group Method to Classification in Philadelphia in May 1932. It was during these meetings that the terms "group therapy" and "group psychotherapy" were defined by Moreno.

In 1957, the International Committee met at the 2nd International Congress of Group Psychotherapy, in Zurich, and made important decisions: the first step was to compose a provisionary council for the future international association. Another matter was to enlarge the membership so as to make the future association more representative. An election would be held by mail ballot to name a new executive committee and a new set of officers. These representatives would write the constitution for the organization.

In Milan, in July of 1963, during the 3rd International Congress of Group Psychotherapy (organized by Enzo Spaltro), the International Council of Group Psychotherapy was founded and, as Anne Ancelin Schützenberger* observed, "group-analysts and psychodramatists [were] together, finally". The election of officers, by mail ballot, had taken place before the Congress. Moreno was made President, with S. H. Foulkes (UK) and Serge Lebovici (France) as Vice-Presidents, Berthold Stokvis (Netherlands), Secretary, and A. Friedemann (Switzerland), Treasurer. In the *International Handbook of Group Psychotherapy* – the proceedings of the 1963 Milan Congress – is the following report:

> Over 100 delegates attended the council meeting. The discussion centered largely on the proposed constitution of the International Association of Group Psychotherapy. Dr. J. L. Moreno opened the discussions and pointed out that only the entire membership of the International Council can make ultimate, binding decisions by anonymous ballot.
>
> The discussion brought out a number of valuable suggestions as to what form the constitution of the International Society should take.
>
> (Moreno, 1966, p. 727)

The 4th International Congress of Group Psychotherapy in Vienna, 1968, was the last congress before the international incorporation. It permitted debate on the developing association. A lively discussion ensued over the structure of the constitution to be adopted. According to Moreno (1968, p. 89), "the range of opinions was wide and most constructive". He added, as President of the International Council, that the task must be completed within a reasonable time and the material circulated. In fact, the final incorporation, five years later, was the result of more than ten years of meetings and correspondence to establish the by-laws. The entire process took more than twenty years, from 1951 until 1973.

At the 5th International Congress of Group Psychotherapy in Zurich, August 19–24, 1973, the long awaited event finally happened. R. Battegay,

A. Friedemann and A. Uchtenhagen organized it, and a comprehensive book on the proceedings of the Congress, under the title *Group Therapy and Social Environment* (Uchtenhagen *et al.*, 1975), was published.

By 1973 Moreno was 84 years old and had suffered several minor strokes. He was not in the best condition to travel, but he insisted on going. It was to be his last international trip and, as Zerka Moreno* pointed out, "Yes, it was J. L.'s very last trip abroad; he died 9 months later. So this was his last baby, so to speak." A few weeks prior to the trip to Zurich, Moreno called his student, translator and friend, Grete Leutz, in Germany, to inform her of his poor physical condition and ask her to find an assistant to help him get around the hotel while Zerka was at the Congress.

There was excitement in the air. The decision that there should be a balance between group analysts and psychodramatists was met on good terms. Candidates for the first executive committee were discussed. Samuel Hadden (USA) was suggested as the first president by the group analysts. Moreno had had some difficulties in the past with Hadden (who was a follower of S. R. Slavson, with whom Moreno had argued over the foundings of group psychotherapy) and would have preferred Adolf Friedemann (Switzerland), but he declined due to a serious heart condition. Despite this, according to Zerka Moreno, considering that Sam Hadden was one of the least offensive opponents, and as a conciliatory gesture regarding that old battle, Moreno agreed and Hadden was designated. Malcolm Pines*, who was there representing S. H. Foulkes, comments that Sam Hadden "was a good choice because he was conscientious and honorable", and remembers that "he used to carry a little pocket book of parliamentary procedures and so every step that we took was legitimate". Adolf Friedemann was made Treasurer–General Secretary. Anne Ancelin Schützenberger (France) was International Secretary, and later International Co-Secretary with Raymond Battegay (Switzerland). Anneliese Heigl-Evers (Germany) was one of the Vice-Presidents. Adolf Friedemann and Raymond Battegay prepared the registration of the institution under Swiss law.

The first session of the international incorporation of the IAGP took place at the Grand Hotel Dolder Berg, in Zurich, in late August 1973. Grete Leutz* describes this memorable day poetically:

> Moreno, sitting at the head of a long table, presided the assembly; at least twelve persons sat by his side. Facing the afternoon sun, he did not speak much, but smiling benevolently, he was very present and appeared satisfied. In the evening he refrained from participating in the second session. Instead, he had dinner with the wife and daughter of Dr. Raoul Schindler (who played an outstanding role in the founding of the IAGP), and me. Inspired by the Viennese voices of the Austrian ladies, he became very spirited and in the most sparkling way, related anecdotes of his time in the literary circles of Vienna . . .

Important people from the group psychotherapy and psychodrama movement were present. Some of them became officers of the association in the years to come, including the four subsequent presidents, Raymond Battegay (Switzerland), Malcolm Pines (UK), Jay Fidler (USA) and Grete Leutz (Germany), and the two next vice-presidents, Anne Ancelin Schützenberger and Zerka Moreno. Also present were Heika Straub (Germany) and Joshua Bierer (UK). Bierer, who sat next to Zerka Moreno, told her that she should have been designated president. Zerka* responded that this would be a mistake because "they obviously wanted both a man and a psychiatrist at the helm". In fact, of the nine elected presidents until now (1997), there have been only two women (Grete Leutz and Fern Cramer Azima), and only two psychologists (Fern Cramer Azima and Earl Hopper) as presidents.

Soon after taking his post as President, Samuel B. Hadden published the following communiqué:

Formation of the International Association of Group Psychotherapy

During the Fifth International Congress of Group Psychotherapy in Zurich in August 1973, a new organization, The International Association of Group Psychotherapy, was formed, a Constitution adopted, and an Interim Board of Directors elected.

   The Constitution provides for National Organizational and Individual memberships to join the planning of future congresses and other measures to advance various forms of Group Psychotherapy. Because of your demonstrated interest, we are inviting you to complete the application and join us at this time.

(Hadden, 1974, p. 240)

J. L. and Zerka Moreno had an active role in all of the first international congresses of group psychotherapy and psychodrama up to 1973, and, obviously, in the foundation of the IAGP. They sometimes even funded the events, as they did with the first three international congresses of group psychotherapy (Toronto, Zurich and Milan). The publication of the *International Handbook of Group Psychotherapy* (1966) co-edited by Battegay and Friedemann, also came out of their own pockets.[1] As Grete Leutz* said: "In all these events, Moreno was the most powerful motor, the 'spiritus rector', and Zerka was totally involved in all those steps."

---

1 Many pioneers put their own money into the first congresses of group psychotherapy and psychodrama. Anne Ancelin Schützenberger, for example, paid the deficit of the 1968 Congress of Psychodrama that was moved from Prague to Baden when the Soviets invaded Czechoslovakia.

A series of coincidences happened in Zurich in late August of 1973. As mentioned earlier, it was Moreno's last international trip and, presumably, his last public presentation. Returning to Beacon, he wrote an open letter that was probably his last published text. He died a few months later (May, 1974). He was passing the baton, conscious that his mission had been fulfilled. We can interpret his words as both a farewell and a request for the continuation of his work, together with the international community of group psychotherapy. This open letter is still relevant today, so I would like to conclude with its transcription. In the contents of *Group Psychotherapy and Psychodrama*, vol. XXVI, no. 3–4 (Moreno, 1973) the following appears: "Open Letter from J. L. Moreno in behalf of the International Association of Group Psychotherapy" (p. 131):

International Association of Group Psychotherapy
Registered under the Swiss Civil Code, Art. 60 ff

Dear Friends:
The newly established International Association of Group Psychotherapy is one of the major goals I have been trying to attain since 1951.
Now that it is a reality, I hope you will give it every support. We need
support of both a moral and financial nature if we are to maintain a
high level of academic pursuit and continued contact at International
Congresses with colleagues all over the world.
    The enclosed membership application is your chance to give evidence
of your interest. It is a crowning achievement of my life's work.

Thank you.
Sincerely yours,
J. L. Moreno, M.D.
Honorary President

References

* Indicates personal correspondence with Raymond Battegay, Juan Campos, Grete Leutz, Zerka Moreno, Malcolm Pines and Anne Ancelin Schützenberger.

Group Psychotherapy (1951) Announcements, vol. IV, nos 1–2 (April–August), p. 126.
Hadden, S. B. (1974). International Association of Group Psychotherapy, *Group Psychotherapy and Psychodrama*, XXVII, 1–4: 240.
Moreno, J. L. (1966). In: J. L. Moreno, A. Friedemann, R. Battegay and Zerka Moreno, *International Handbook of Group Psychotherapy*. New York: Philosophical Library.

Moreno, J. L. (1968). Open Letter to the Members of the International Council of Group Psychotherapy. *Group Psychotherapy*, XXI, 2–3 (June–September): 89.

Moreno, J. L. (1973). Open Letter from J. L. Moreno in behalf of the International Association of Group Psychotherapy. *Group Psychotherapy and Psychodrama*, XXVI, 3–4: 131.

Moreno, Z. T. (1954). International Committee on Group Psychotherapy and the First International Congress on Group Psychotherapy, *Group Psychotherapy*, 7, 1: 91.

Uchtenhagen, A., Battegay, R. and Friedemann, A. (1975). *Group Therapy and Social Environment*. Proceedings of the 5th International Congress for Group Psychotherapy, Bern/Stuttgart/Wien: Hans Huber Publishers.

Additional works consulted

Audio-tape interview with Zerka Moreno by Juan Campos in Barcelona, October 31, 1988.

Marineau, R. F. (1989). *Jacob Levy Moreno 1889–1974. Father of psychodrama, sociometry and group psychotherapy*. London/New York: Tavistock/Routledge.

Moreno, Z. T. (1966). Evolution and dynamics of the group psychotherapy movement. In: J. L. Moreno, A. Friedemann, R. Battegay and Zerka Moreno, *The International Handbook of Group Psychotherapy*. New York: Philosophical Library, pp. 27–125.

Schützenberger, A. A. (1970). Breve histórico do psicodrama na França (A brief history of psychodrama in France). In: *O teatro da vida: psicodrama*. São Paulo: Livraria Duas Cidades, pp. 217–223.

Schützenberger, A. A. (1970). *Introducción al psicodrama (Introduction to psychodrama)*. Madrid: Aguilar. (Original edition: *Precis de Psychodrame. Introduction aux Aspectos Techniques*. Paris: Editions Universitaires, 1966.)

Schützenberger, A. A. (1978). *Introdução à dramatização (Introduction to dramatization)*. Belo Horizonte: Interlivros. (Original edition: *Introduction au jeu de rôle*. Paris: Edoaurd Privat, Editeur, 1975.)

Note: Thanks to Grete Leutz, Zerka Moreno, Anne Ancelin Schützenberger and David Kipper for their contributions and their kindness.

Chapter 15

Tendencies in psychotherapy and the role of psychodrama

I come from a part of the world with quite different cultural connotations. The Brazilian psychodramatic movement has had a rather different history from other parts of the world, as mentioned in the Introduction. J. L. Moreno predicted in 1961 that Latin culture would be fertile ground for the growth of psychodrama, and he was right; indeed, there are approximately 4,000 people working with psychodrama in Brazil and our biannual congresses attract roughly 1,000 participants. It is, therefore, from this cultural background that my comments originate – though I also consider information that I have gathered through my work with the IAGP (International Association of Group Psychotherapy).

I would like to point out some of the historical highlights of psychotherapy, group psychotherapy and psychodrama so that we can better understand the present and contemplate the future.

Psychoanalysis

Every revolutionary must be an extremist in order to reach his/her objectives – just look at examples from history – and Freud certainly was, especially in regard to his theory of sexuality. While modern sex studies have confirmed many Freudian proposals, they have refuted others, such as those referring to female sexuality (a woman's orgasm is either clitoral or vaginal, the former being immature or infantile and the latter mature) and masturbation (which Freud claimed would lead to hysteria and psychasthenia). The psychoanalytic groundwork (etiology) of psychotic profiles is still questioned even today. The idea that latent homosexuality in itself could lead to paranoia is also arguable. In short, many Freudian *truths* have lost their validity, just as many current *truths* will fall by the wayside. All the same, among the hits and misses, disagreements and exaggerations, psychoanalysis has transcended medicine and psychology, impregnating twentieth-century culture.

The 1940s and 1950s marked the zenith of psychoanalytic ideas (in Brazil, this phenomenon came about more in the 1950s and 1960s).

Everything became "psychological" – *psychocentrism* – and "sexual" – *sexcentrism*. Various diseases of unknown origin such as collagen diseases (lupus, rheumatoid arthritis), peptic ulcers, psoriasis, vitiligo, etc. were considered to have possible psychological roots. From the psychodynamic explanation of forgetfulness and deceptions to the psychoanalytic view toward neuroses and psychoses, everything became subject to the interpretation: "Freud can explain it." While on the one hand, this divulgation served to democratize the psychoanalytic language, it also motivated interpretative exaggeration. The culture became psychological and interpretative, leading to *interpretosis*. Biological methods and treatments, such as chemical and electroshock therapies, were abhorred. The image of neuropsychiatric surgery was blemished due to the indiscriminate performance of lobotomies, the fruit of previous trends. This exaggerated criticism was worth while, however, as it ushered in changes in psychiatry. Also in the 1950s, neuroleptics came on the scene – first chlorpromazine, followed by levopromazine, then haloperidol – which fostered a revolution in psychiatry, a true second coming of the mental illnesses (the first having been promoted by Pinel).

"Organicism", "psychologism" and the old paradigms

The clash of forces at the beginning of the twentieth century between the *organistic* and psychodynamic currents in psychiatry continues now between the biochemical and psychological lines. The *emotionalization* of this dispute includes struggles for power and marketing advantages. However, above all else it reflects a human characteristic: competitiveness. This, like other human traits, has its positive and negative sides. Positive competition propels progress. It respects contrary arguments, reverses roles with the opposition and is never ruled by fanaticism. Under these circumstances, the certainty that truth is relative, not absolute, and that one cannot see the parts without the whole, predominates. Descartes criticized the medieval scholastic philosophers who used the sterile *disputative* method, in which one argued similarly in favor or against anything, with no decisive defense for either position. Aristotle defined *apaideusia* as the "lack of education in the sense of lack of instruction, someone wanting to have the same degree of certainty in all areas of knowledge" (Nascimento, 1995, p. 25).

The organic/psychic dichotomy of the *organistic* and psychodynamic psychiatrists at the beginning of the twentieth century started to dilute when psychoanalytic ideas became absorbed by the culture. In the United States, the *dynamic psychiatry* movement appeared at the end of the 1940s, reflected in Argentina and Brazil in the 1960s and 1970s (the book *Dynamic Psychiatry* by Franz Alexander was published in America in 1947 and in Argentina in 1958). This current put forth a psychodynamic approach toward mental illness, in which both organic and psychological aspects were taken into account. In this period, a balance of power between these two approaches began, resulting in a crop of clinical psychiatrists with psychodynamic instruction. As a witness to this period (at the State Public Service Hospital and the Clinical Hospital in São Paulo), as both a student and professor, I recall that the emphasis in psychiatric training was broad and homogeneous. We could be, or rather we were supposed to be, clinical psychiatrists and psychotherapists. Nowadays, due to the advances in neuropsychobiological[1] research, we have returned to the dichotomy in which representatives from these opposing currents do not overlap their functions, display rivalrous conduct and view each other with distrust. Mutual ignorance is responsible for embarrassing situations where psychotherapeutic psychiatrists prescribe drugs erroneously (due to ignorance of psychopharmacology) and clinical psychiatrists relate disastrously to patients and their families (due to lack of relational sensitivity). Perhaps it really is impossible, now, to perform these two functions with the same competence, but certainly a more flexible relationship between the two is possible.

Attempts to overcome the scientific differences of the twentieth century, despite all good intentions, have not produced great results. Since the time I began my medical studies, quite some time ago, I have repeatedly heard that we must have a bio-psycho-social focus toward illness, but this has become a more theoretical than practical enunciation. Not that there is ill will in following this beautiful pronouncement. Rather, it is due more to the difficulty in putting this into practice under current scientific paradigms. The same could be said of interdisciplinarity – none is opposed, everyone in favor. But, in truth, what interdisciplinarity really exists in our universities? I was recently told that, during a discussion on interdisciplinarity at a certain university, one participant recalled that the only thing connecting the various departments was the campus shuttle bus!

I believe that many of our dilemmas would be considerably alleviated if a broader view toward human phenomena were adopted. Just as was once believed in astronomy, it may be that we still believe, in psychiatry, that the earth is flat or that the sun revolves around the earth, the center of the universe. Careful analysis reveals that both *organicism* and *psychologism* are based on the same parameters which ruled all the sciences during this period. I refer to the Cartesian paradigm of the mind–body division and to Newtonian *causalistic* determinism. The conception that the universe is a

---

1 Starting in the 1960s, in terms of physiopathological concepts, there was a shift from the simplistic belief that mental illnesses had no apparent physical cause to the "neurotransmitter era", then to the "receptor era", and finally to the current "molecular era".

great *machine* ruled by mechanical laws that determine all the causes of all phenomena has been wholly accepted in medicine. Man has come to be seen as a machine whose parts wear out, needing removal or repair. Added to this is the imperialism of mathematical certainty that has impregnated all twentieth century science. It is as if only "hard" science brings forth truths while "soft" science remains dubious.

Despite the fact that physics has transcended the Cartesian and mechanistic posture, evolving toward new paradigms, there is a resistance in medicine and psychology toward these new references. In truth, the *reductionist/divisionist* concept, in having brought and continuing to bring spectacular progress, remains very seductive. Medicine in the future will continue dividing man, no longer organ by organ but gene by gene. There is an insistence in denying that, even if this model is beneficial for the development of certain areas in medicine, it is innocuous for others. No one questions the great advances made in medicine from the discovery of the correlation between bacteria and illness, or from the appearance of antibiotics, or from the evolution of surgical techniques. However, it is also known that the majority of people who have been equally exposed to the same bacteria do not fall ill, others who have received antibiotics do not respond to them, and that many patients who were operated on in one decade would not be in another. For example, the performance of tonsillectomies in the 1950s and 1960s, of gastrectomies in the 1960s and 1970s and of coronary implants (safena and mammary points) in the 1970s and 1980s was much more prevalent at those times than now, indicating that *scientific* recommendations are also subject to trends. Likewise, until very recently, doctors attempted to hide from their cancer patients that they had the disease. It was believed that such news would drive the patient to desperation, even suicide. Today the order is to tell all, even things the patient doesn't want to hear. I recently had a patient in psychotherapy who denied to his death that he had Aids, despite all evidence and information to the contrary. Wouldn't it be more practical to provide training to medical students to improve their ability to perceive what a patient wants to know about his/her state of health?

The field of medicine is much broader than that proposed by traditional medicine, but this ignorance stems not from the doctors themselves but rather from the culture at large. For example, in the West, a doctor's success in his/her private clinic is measured by the number of ill people he/she sees. In China, this signifies a professional disaster. There, a good doctor is one who prevents his/her patients from becoming ill in the first place. Here, the emphasis is on curative medicine, while there, on preventive medicine. The Japanese approach organ transplants with reservation, as the body and soul are considered to be one unit, as are man and nature.

For a better understanding of modern medicine, a few historical facts from American medicine, the leader of all Western medicine (including, obviously, ours in Brazil), must be recalled. The current biomedical model is the fruit of the Flexner Report, published in 1910, which served as the basis for the reformulation of American medical education. The report was made in response to a solicitation from the American Medical Association, in the hopes of both improving the quality of education and channeling funds from recently established foundations (among them the Rockefeller and Carnegie Foundations) to medical schools. This fact established a partnership between medicine and American big business (including the pharmaceutical and medical equipment industries) "which has come to dominate, until today, the entire health care system" (Capra, 1988, p. 151). The result of this policy has been *reductionist* medicine, in the biological sense, with fewer general practitioners and more specialists, more complementary exams and recommendations for surgery, in addition to the excessive prescription of medications. Attending gravely ill and hospitalized patients has become more valued than common or outpatient cases, ignoring the fact that these are the great majority in clinical practice. This biomedical model has reached the status of dogma, going unquestioned by medical practitioners.

The Cartesian–Newtonian biomedical approach, despite its undeniable utility, is insufficient for the comprehension of all human suffering. The greatest leap in science in general, and in medicine in particular, will happen when a different philosophy is adopted. Still in the twentieth century, a few attempts to supplant the old scientific structures were made, among them systemic theory, constructivism and holism. Even if these were unable to provoke the revolution intended, they at least offered new approaches to human phenomena. They broke away from the linear, deterministic, *unicausal* focus and presented the concepts of circularity and feedback. That is, component A may affect component B; B may affect C; and C may feed back to A, thus closing the circuit. When a system is interrupted there are multiple causes since they feed each other reciprocally, making the search for a single cause of failure irrelevant. Capra transposes these concepts to medicine, saying "this state of non-linear interconnection of living organisms indicates that the conventional attempts of biomedical science to associate illness with a single cause are problematic. Furthermore, it shows the failure of 'genetic determinism'" (Capra, 1988, p. 262). The systemic perspective makes clear that genes are not the exclusive determinants of an organism's function, like gears determine the functioning of a watch. Genes are, however, integral parts of an ordered whole which, therefore, can be adapted to a systemic organization.

Psychology, as it couldn't fail to be, was also molded on the same Cartesian–Newtonian dichotomy, resulting in the same ambiguities found in the biomedical model. The two great psychological currents at the beginning of the century, behaviorism and psychoanalysis, are based on the mechanistic, deterministic, *causalist* model. Behaviorism, which generated behavioral and cognitive therapies, reduces human behavior to a mechanical sequence of conditioned responses. Psychoanalysis, in the same way, is seated in the laws of physics, especially mechanical, hydraulic and thermodynamic. In this way, Freud explains all psychological and psychopathological manifestations according to a linear chain of cause and effect. Everything that was biological to the organicist becomes psychological to the psychoanalyst. *Theories* explaining everything are faced with reservation. There is an excess of *because* and a lack of *how*.

Moreno presents psychodrama as an alternative to these two methodologies:

> Behavioristic schools have been limited to observing and experimenting with "external" behavior of individuals, leaving out major portions of the subjective. Many psychological methods, such as psychoanalysis . . . went to the other extreme, focusing on the subjective but limiting the study of direct behavior to a minimum and resorting to the use of elaborate systems of symbolic interpretation.
>
> (Moreno, 1977, p. xxi)

Jonathan D. Moreno (1989) adds that his father's "behaviorism" was more similar to that of George Herbert Mead and John Dewey than to that of John Watson or B. F. Skinner. I believe that Moreno's "behaviorism" is actually more *strategic* than behavioural.

Recognizing the limitations of the twentieth-century psychotherapies doesn't mean tarnishing their creators and followers. On the contrary, all of this was good, even if it is insufficient. A *reductionist* description may be useful and, in some cases, necessary: "It is only dangerous when interpreted as if it were a complete description. Reductionism and holism, analysis and synthesis, are complementary focuses which, when used in the appropriate balance, help us reach a deeper understanding" (Capra, 1988, p. 116).

Psychodrama and the new paradigms[2]

Much of the criticism of Moreno's work refers to the fact that it was considered intuitive, in detriment to a logical, rational line, overly emphasized the description of the *whole* to the analysis of the parts, and didn't explain mental illness in terms of cause and effect. Attempts to supplant the old *reductionist* models are frequently labeled as superficial and inconsistent. There is something strange about seeing the world without the old

---

2 I make use of the texts of Seixas (1992), Tozoni-Reis (1992), Castello de Almeida (1994), Figueiredo (1996) and Landini (1998) who discuss the place of psychodrama in scientific methodology.

linear, causal paradigms. Gestalt therapy and psychodrama are included within this new model. The Spanish psychiatrist Pablo Poblacion (1992) said:

> We are attempting a systems approach of psychodrama . . . For many years we have defended that Moreno was a pioneer of systems theory in the field of social structures, which he denominated in a way that globalized "socionomics" . . . The paradigm of the Morenian systems position is in its concepts, currently much debated, that there is no role without a counter-role; that a role originates in a relationship, later configuring relationships; that the family is a unit and must be treated as such, etc.
>
> (Poblacion, 1992, p. 146)

If one considers the fact that Moreno's work was written almost entirely in the first half of the twentieth century, when the scientific paradigms opposed his methodology – that is, preached the analysis of the parts and causality in the study of phenomena – the difficulties he faced in implementing his ideas can be understood.

In his first work, a poem called "Invitation to an Encounter" (Einladung zu einer Begegnung, Anzengruber Verlag, Vienna, 1914), Moreno makes his relational viewpoint clear. This now famous passage is part of it: "A meeting of two: eye to eye, face to face/And when you are near I will tear your eyes out/and place them instead of mine/and you will tear my eyes out/ and will place them instead of yours/then I will look at you with your eyes/ and you will look at me with mine . . ."

In *The Words of the Father* ([1920] 1971), Moreno introduces a surprising view of the hierarchical relationship of man to God. Consistent with the Hasidic influences he received, he presents a creator–creation relationship structured upon mutual dependence – a horizontal relationship, where both poles are essential to the balance of the system. God would be nothing without man, who would be nothing without God. God and man are co-creators: the former is the director and the latter the auxiliary ego in the psychodrama of life. Moreno goes further, bringing the possibility of God to the first person: the Creativity God, the God in me, the I–God. Also in *The Words of the Father*, Moreno foreshadows systemic theory:

> How can one thing/create another thing/unless the other thing/creates the one thing?/How can a first thing/create a second thing/unless the second thing/also creates the first?/How can a second thing/create a third thing/unless the third thing/also creates the second?/How can a third thing/create a fourth thing/unless the fourth thing/also creates the third?/How can a father beget a son/unless the son/also begets his father?/How can a grandfather/beget a grandson/unless the grandson is

a/grandfather to his grandfather?/The first created the last/and the end created the beginning./I created the world/therefore must I have created myself.

(Moreno, [1920] 1971, p. 53)

In *The Theater of Spontaneity* (1924), after observing the actors' spontaneous role performances, Moreno revealed the possibility of training spontaneity. He was concerned with the fact that spontaneity could become *rancorous*, becoming *spontaneism*, meaning an erroneous creative route. This led him to the search for techniques for developing *healthy* spontaneity: the spontaneous theater, the live newspaper, psychomusic, psychodance, role-play and psychodrama.

In *Who Shall Survive?* (1994 [1934]), Moreno makes an effort to prove, according to the scientific criteria of that time, that humanity is composed of groups ruled by sociodynamic laws, according to forces of attraction, repulsion and neutrality. Group structures comprise isolated individuals, pairs, triangles, circles, networks, stars, sociometric leaders, social atoms, chains, psychological currents, etc. These configurations can be learned (measured) by a sociometric test and mapped into sociograms.

In 1946, Moreno at last presented a new psychotherapeutic method, consistent with his previous philosophical ideas, in *Psychodrama I* (followed by *Psychodrama II* and *III*). The main objective of this new psychotherapeutic approach was not to analyze the patient according to the linear criteria of symptom cause and effect – though this could eventually happen – but rather to free the patient's spontaneity, strangled by the personal and interpersonal conflicts which the individual had experienced throughout his/her lifetime.

If I were asked to choose the most important element of Morenian theory I would select the relational focus of his philosophy. This relational aspect appears in all his concepts, be it role theory (role and counter-role), the concepts of tele-relationship and the encounter, in sociometry, the identity matrix (the child's first relational network), and so on. For Moreno, humanity comprises a network of apparent and subjacent relationships interacting. The *social tricotomy* is made up of the tangible, external society, by the *sociometric matrix* – the sociometric structure invisible to macroscopic observation, and by the *social reality*, the synthesis of the two. Perhaps the following citation by Moreno himself best explains the relational focus of psychodrama theory:

If we observe the universe, we see life among its interconnected organisms, in an interdependent state; if we look, with particular attention, at the organisms that inhabit the earth, we can note two aspects of this interdependent state: a horizontal or geographic structure and a vertical structure. We can also observe that the most highly differentiated organisms need and depend on the less differentiated. It is this order of heterogeneous things that makes bacteria and algae indispensable to more complex structures, which couldn't exist without them; it is this order that permits the survival of creatures so vulnerable and dependent as man.

(Moreno, 1994, p. 91)

Moreno had antennae, an intuition for new paradigms, and tried to orient his work within them. However, he lacked the appropriate language for the simple reason that it didn't exist during his time – it was the language of the future that he barely lived to see (he died in 1974). Though he captured the transformations, he was imprecise in expressing them. In the natural succession of scientific paradigms, he announced a new paradigm, but was obligated to use the old language.[3] Moreno was ahead of his time. He was a visionary, in the sense of one who has a vision – a *pre-vision* – of the future.

Capra (1988) discusses the transformation of scientific criteria. He proposes the transformation of assertive values into integrative values: of the rational to the intuitive, the fragmented to the holistic, the linear to the non-linear, domination to partnership. This new vision of reality "is based on the consciousness of the inter-related and interdependent state essential to all physical, biological, social and cultural phenomena" (Capra, 1988, p. 259). Within this thinking, although "we can discern individual parts in any system, the nature of the whole is always different than the mere sum of the parts" (ibid., p. 261).

Also according to Capra, the basic proposals of systems theory thinking are: (1) the whole is greater than the sum of the parts; (2) to understand the whole, the *relationships* of the parts among themselves in their different possible combinations must be taken into account; (3) as a result of these two items, knowledge, formerly given as the objective, becomes instead relational and contextual; (4) instead of questioning the content, con-figurations of relationships that repeat themselves – that is, become a model – are observed; (5) a model cannot be measured or weighed, but can be mapped (quality overrides quantity); (6) the notion of hierarchy comes to be viewed through the network in which it is constituted; (7) to the extent that life is approached as the dynamic configuration of the components of its whole, the energy which flows throughout the system is recognized and one can speak of a process of living structures.

3 Up to now, the following paradigms can be denominated: Copernican, Cartesian, Darwinian and systemic. The appearance of a new scientific paradigm will happen in the third millennium.

The relational view of psychodrama is absolutely correlated to systemic theory. The focus of both even coincides: networks, relationships, models, processes, mapping, etc.

> To see from a systems approach is to see psychodramatically, is to put oneself within the context, perceiving the parts, the relationships, the models, without losing sight of the whole, accompanying the processes in a flexible and dynamic way, understanding the oscillation of opposites and knowing oneself to be one with the universe.
>
> (Figueiredo, 1996, p. 6)

Group era

The fusion of the psychological with the social began with the studies developed on group dynamics during the Second World War. The 1960s and 1970s marked the *group era*. Psychoanalytic group psychotherapy, group analysis, psychodrama, the person-centered approach, and gestalt therapy came to emphasize the group approach. In the United States, two locations were prominent in spreading the group movement: Beacon, with the World Center of Psychodrama led by J. L. Moreno, and Bethel, with the NTL (National Training Laboratory) led by Kurt Lewin. Later, the Esalen Institute also became distinguished as a group and alternative therapy temple. This dynamic peak of group psychotherapy coincided with the hippie culture and its communal life proposal.

This period also marked the advent of anti-psychiatry, initiated by Ronald Laing and David Cooper in England. As stated previously, all revolutions – or attempts at revolution – contain extremism. While anti-psychiatry may have sinned from an excess of romanticism, in which "going crazy" gained the contours of self-development and the socio-familiar was, supposedly, the cause of insanity (this was at least an advance in terms of the former schizophrenogenic mother theory), it also contributed to the humanization of psychiatric hospitals, helped reduce prejudice toward mental illness and opened the doors to family psychotherapy. Anti-psychiatry was the precursor to the disputed Italian psychiatric revolution promoted by Franco Basaglia.

The narcissistic cultural syndrome of the end of the twentieth century

In the 1980s, within the middle and upper social classes generically, a "culture of the individual" arose from the internal growth achieved through individual meditative practices and from the cult of beauty and health. A sophisticated style of living was proposed, and great financial maneuvers, often accomplished with merely a click on a keyboard, exalted. It was the kingdom of the clean, the prevalence of *I* over *us*, the *me decade*. It dealt with the yuppie as opposed to the hippie. The individual replaced the group and the private substituted the public. Communities and dormitories were replaced by small individual apartments. Group psychotherapy was left behind for individual therapy or simply "taking our Prozac every day". Cleanliness, order and beauty became the idealized goals. Long, unkempt hair was cut and controlled with gel. Even if, on the one hand, this cultural movement put forth some healthy habits, on the other hand, in its exaggeration, it revealed hypochondriac and narcissistic features. One must not forget that a psychological reading of Nazism means the narcissistic ideal of purity, perfection, beauty and superiority. Coincidentally or not, in the political arena, a resurgence of the right could be observed, reflected in various areas of human activity. An apparent conservatism also impregnated the sciences. It is within this greater scientific–cultural context that psychiatry and psychotherapy must be situated. Everything indicates that the *neo-organicism* or biochemistry of current psychiatry was placed within this new world order of values. It is within this scientific–cultural syndrome that we live: the narcissistic cultural syndrome of the end of the century.

In this context, we arrive at the *cerebral decade*. President Clinton and the American Congress named the 1990s as such, in the sense of emphasizing the increase in research into cerebral physiology and physiopathology. A new phase and – why not? – a new mode in psychiatry began: the biochemical justification to explain psychopathological profiles and personality traits. Thus, as in the past, everything that was organic and then psychological became biochemical or genetic. Sfez (1996) says ironically that it is as if we have the *devil within the body*: genes for depression, drug addiction and, who knows? – maybe even for homelessness.

Perspectives on psychotherapies for the twenty-first century

The dispute between the *psychological camp* and the *biochemical or organistic camp* in psychiatry will continue despite the fact that neurosciences and psychology are beginning a dialogue. It is easy to suggest that we maintain an "ideal" attitude – that of emotional absence – in considering these two camps. But, beyond being unrealistic, this wouldn't allow for the positive channeling of constructive energies, which can only occur when these feelings are brought to consciousness. As Forbes (1996, p. 5) says: "Between psychodynamics and psychiatry, there is a dialectic tension with benefit to both when their agents permit themselves to be questioned, which, unfortunately, is not always the case."

We can also expect the discovery of the genetic components of some mental illnesses and personality characteristics; this will lead to a reappraisal of their psychosocial aspects and, as a consequence, a re-evaluation of their psychotherapeutic management. There will be a reduction in the number of indiscriminate referrals to psychotherapy, resulting in fewer professionals in the area of psychology.

Psychoanalysis, linked to the International Psychoanalytic Association (IPA) and other related nuclei, will represent the orthodoxy responsible for research into the unconscious, not solely concerned with the psychotherapeutic aspect of this practice. Orthodox psychoanalysis will have an elitist posture, necessary for the preservation of Freudian principles and for the supply of subsidies to psychodynamic psychotherapies. Psychoanalysts who hope to survive financially will have to make their practice more flexible, especially in respect to the number of weekly sessions demanded: four or five weekly sessions will become history. The new psychotherapeutic schools, even those inspired by psychoanalysis, will avoid the *old* paradigms focused on the penis and breast, seeking broader ones. There will be a tendency to merge the elements found in the laboratory and on the couch.

Psychotherapy, in a generic sense, as a practice that purports to help people with psychological suffering, will adapt to the new scientific cultural and economic order. Within this new order there is a trend toward methods with proven results. This is a pressure that, despite protest, will install objectivity in psychotherapy. Concerning objectivity and speed, the ample use of strategic and action techniques (cognitive psychotherapy, psychotherapy, gestalt therapy and neurolinguistic programming, among others) is predicted. In addition, techniques that employ altered states of consciousness, such as internal psychodrama (psychotherapeutic work with internally visualized images) and the various hypnosis and autosuggestion techniques (Ericksonian psychotherapy, for example), will become more greatly appreciated.

We mustn't forget recent advances in the study of brain functioning and the increasing correlation between neuroscience (the brain) and psychology (the mind). It is particularly interesting to observe that a child's developing brain can be seen as an interpersonal phenomenon. Brain structures do not provide the only means by which we relate to others, as relational experience fosters brain development. In other words, the stimulation which comes from the primary social relationship (identity matrix) is indispensable to continued brain growth.

One could say that spontaneity flows between two (or more) people (in this case, child and caretaker) just as flows between neurons in the brain. The orbitofrontal cortex, wired to reach facial expressions and particularly sensitive to face-to-face communication, may also play an important role in the development of *telic sensitivity* or the capacity for empathy in the future adult.

These advances in interpersonal neurobiology open the doors to a conceptual bridge between biology and relationship psychology which will change the theoretical and practical posture of psychotherapies. As comprehension of the main and secondary personality traits and their respective symptoms improves as a result of this linkage, psychotherapeutic techniques will undoubtedly become more efficient in this century.

We will witness the union of Western psychotherapeutic techniques with those from the East such as meditation, visualization and the broadening of consciousness. There will also be the fusion of cybernetic techniques such as biofeedback (for example, the person visualizes his/her blood pressure and learns how to control it) and the *PET scan* (*positron emission tomography* – when one is able, for example, to visualize the light in the arteries) with Eastern relaxation and internal visualization techniques. This type of focus has every chance of being employed in the psychotherapeutic approach to functional and organic pathologies in various medical specialties. Carl Simonton – in oncology – and Dean Ornish – in cardiology – have initiated a medical movement which will only tend to grow: the introduction of psychotherapy (both individual and group) and internal visualization techniques as co-actors in traditional medical procedures.

Family psychotherapy, which belongs to the group therapy field and includes couples therapy and other related psychotherapies (with different intrafamily sociometric arrangements), will continue developing greatly, due to the direct nature of its approach and the brevity (according to some schools of thought) of its process. Generational research will include genetic and psychological aspects when studying the family profile and the personalities of its members.

The IAGP (International Association of Group Psychotherapy) noted a considerable decrease in the affiliation of new entities to the association in the 1990s, as compared to the 1970s. This suggests that either the groups who intended to join did so in previous years, or, more probably, the group psychotherapy movement no longer presents the same power as before. In the city of São Paulo, there are fewer psychoanalytic and psychodramatic process groups (groups that meet weekly with the same psychotherapist over an extended period) than in the 1970s and 1980s. This has not happened due to a belief that group therapy is a less effective therapy. It continues to be as effective as ever. Rather, it means that process group psychotherapy goes, as we see, against the current cultural tide. The *narcissistic cultural syndrome* of the end of the century opposes the group, the public and the community. In the meantime, the employment of group techniques in workshops, retreats, demonstrations of techniques, courses, and the selection and training of personnel, continues to grow. I think that, in the twenty-first century, group therapies, along with the resulting tendencies mentioned above, will receive the strategic focus of brief and theme (obese groups, phobic groups, etc.) psychotherapies. Group therapies will continue to be useful in community outreach programs directed toward preventive medicine and public health. Individual psychotherapy provides the exclusivity and coziness which group therapy does not. But group psychotherapy offers what individual therapy cannot: relational insertion in a group network and observation through the multiple therapeutic eyes of the group. Individual and group therapy make the psychotherapeutic process complete.

As cultural movements occur in waves, filtered by the values of the time, it is possible that we will have a new *group era*. It may appear as a reaction against the values reminiscent of the yuppies and the narcissistic cultural syndrome of the end of the century. It would be a neo-hippie phase. We would have a new-found appreciation of the group, of the community and of the group psychotherapy process. But I am not sure if this is a prediction or the desire of the author who misses the values of his youth.

References

Alexander, F. (1947). *Dynamic psychiatry*. Chicago: The University of Chicago Press.

Capra, F. (1988). *O ponto de mutação*. São Paulo: Cultrix. (Original edition: *The turning point*. New York: Simon & Schuster, 1982.)

Castello de Almeida, W. (1994). O lugar do psicodrama (The place of psychodrama). In: S. Petrilli, *Rosa dos ventos da teoria do psicodrama. (The theory of psychodrama pinwheel)*. São Paulo: Ágora.

Figueiredo, M. (1996). Caminho para aprendizagem psicodramatica (The way to psychodramatic learning). Sociedade de Psicodrama de São Paulo.

Forbes, J. (1996). *Balanço da psicanálise (An evaluation of psychoanalysis)* (booklet). São Paulo.

Landini, J. C. (1998) *Do animal ao humano (From the animal to the human)*. São Paulo: Ágora.

Moreno, J. D. (1989). Introduction in the autobiography of J. L. Moreno. *Journal of Psychotherapy, Psychodrama and Sociometry*, 42, 1 (Spring).

Moreno, J. L. (1920). Das Testament Des Vaters (The Words of the Father). Berlin: Gustav Kiepenheur Verlag.

Moreno, J. L. (1924) Das Stegreiftheater (The Theatre of Spontaneity). Berlin: Gustav Kiepenheur Verlag.

Moreno, J. L. ([1920] 1971). *The words of the Father*. New York: Beacon House, Inc.

Moreno, J. L. (1976). *Psicodrama*. São Paulo: Cultrix. (Original edition: *Psychodrama – First Volume*. New York: Beacon House, Inc., 1946.)

Moreno, J. L. (1977). *Psychodrama – First Volume* (5th edn). New York: Beacon House, Inc.

Moreno, J. L. (1992). *Psicodrama*. São Paulo: Cultrix. (Original edition: *Psychodrama – First Volume*. New York: Beacon House, Inc., 1946.)

Moreno, J. L. (1994). Quem sobreviverá? Goiâna: Dimensão (Original edition: Who shall survive? Washington, DC: Nervous and Mental Diseases Publishing Co., 1934.)

Nascimento, C. A. R. (1995). Monismo e pluralismo epistemologico (Epistemologic monism and pluralism). In: M. L. Martinelli, *O uno e o multiplo (The single and the multiple)*. São Paulo: Cortez.

Poblacion, P. (1992). Metadrama: o metamodelo em psicodrama (Metadrama: the metamodel in psychodrama). *Tema*, 22, 44 (July–December).

Seixas, M. R. (1992). *Sociodrama familiar sistêmico (Systemic family sociodrama)*. São Paulo: Aleph.

Sfez, L. (1996). A grande saúde ("Great" health). Interview for the *Folha de São Paulo*, July 4.

Tozoni-Reis, J. R. (1992). *Cenas familiares (Familiar scenes)*. São Paulo: Ágora.

Wylie, M. S. and Simon, R. (2002). Discoveries from the Black Box – How the neuroscience revolution can change our practice. *Psychotherapy Networker – The Magazine for Today's Helping Professional*.
http://www.psychotherapynetworker.org/black_box.htm.

Index

Note: page numbers in **bold** refer to diagrams.